Published by
Medical Research Modernization Committee

Printed in the United States of America

For information, contact the Medical Research Modernization Committee, Box 2751 Grand Central Station, New York, NY 10163-2751.

Library of Congress National Serials Data Program
International Standard Serial Number 1053-8984

ISBN 0-9623858-8-3 (casebound)
ISBN 0-9623858-9-1 (paperback)

Perspectives on Medical Research
Volume 4, 1993

Edited by

Stephen R. Kaufman
Kathryn Hahner

Published by the Medical Research Modernization Committee

Contents

Essays

Preface

This volume of the *Perspectives* series reports research on the efficacy of different research modalities. As in previous editions, there are several reviews of animal models of human diseases. Expanding on previous research of animal models of childhood diseases, Eric Dunayer evaluates a new animal model of Duchenne muscular dystrophy, and he analyses animal models of two other major genetic childhood diseases--cystic fibrosis and sickle cell anemia. Similarly, Stephen Kaufman, adding to previous work, critiques visual deprivation research on animals and an animal model of orbital floor fractures.

Murry Cohen has reviewed three research projects involving neurology and psychopharmacology. One paper, with three co-authors, addresses controversial experiments on vocalization in monkeys at Northwestern University.

Paul Contard reports exciting developments using a new *in vitro* system to study various tissues, particular skin. Five book reviews covering a broad range of topics related to medical research complete this edition.

Because the MRMC plans to concentrate on disseminating its findings to date, there will be a hiatus in the publication of future volumes of *Perspectives*. Book reviews and analyses of research will appear in our newsletter *MRMC Report*.

Biographical Information on Contributors

Deborah N. Black, M.D., F.R.C.P.(C.)

Dr. Black is a Clinical Instructor at the University of Montréal. She received a B.A. from Vassar College and an M.D.C.M. from McGill University in 1979. She did a residency in neurology at the Montreal Neurological Institute and received an M.Sc. from the McGill University Department of Neurology and Neurosurgery. She is certified by the American Board of Neurology. She has 13 publications and scientific meeting presentations on neurological diseases and two presentations on medical ethical issues.

Murry J. Cohen, M.D.

Dr. Cohen was an Assistant Professor Clinical Psychiatry at Mount Sinai School of Medicine from 1977-1985, and he is currently in private practice. He received a B.A. in psychology from Lehigh University and an M.D. from Chicago Medical School. He did two years of medical training at Montefiore Hospital in the Bronx and completed a residency in psychiatry at Mount Sinai Hospital in New York City. He has published extensively in the areas of drug and alcohol abuse. He is Co-Chair of the Medical Research Modernization Committee.

Paul C. Contard, M.D., Ph.D.

Dr. Contard is on the faculty of the Staten Island University Hospital Department of Medicine. He received a B.A. from Brooklyn College of CUNY in 1980, a Ph.D. from City University of New York in 1987, and an M.D. from Mount Sinai School of Medicine in 1988. He did a dermatology residency and research fellowship at Mount Sinai School of Medicine. He has 12 publications, including several recent articles on a keratinocyte-fibroblast co-culture model.

Frank W. Dobbs, Ph.D.

Dr. Dobbs is a Professor of Chemistry at Northeastern Illinois University. He received his B.A. and M.S. at University of Chicago and his Ph.D. at Massachusetts Institute of Technology. He served as Chair of the Northeastern Illinois University Department of Chemistry from 1971 to 1977 and the Dean of Arts and Sciences from 1977 to 1989. He has written several papers in chemistry and physics and his books include *The Physical Sciences* and *The Age of the Molecule*.

Eric Dunayer, V.M.D.

Dr. Dunayer received his B.A. in biology from the University of Pennsylvania, an M.S. in Environmental Health and Sciences from Drexel University, and a V.M.D. from the University of Pennsylvania. A practicing veterinarian, Dr. Dunayer has written and spoken widely on alternatives to the harmful use of nonhuman animals in research, education, and testing.

Roger S. Fouts, Ph.D.

Dr. Fouts is a Professor in the Department of Psychology at Central Washington University and the Director of the Chimpanzee and Human Communication Institute at Central Washington University. He received a B.A. is psychology from California State College at Long Beach in 1965 and a Ph.D. in experimental psychology for the University of Nevada at Reno in 1971. He has published extensively in the area of non-human primate communication, including work with Project Washoe at the University of Nevada. In addition to consulting to several professional organizations and non-professional publications, he was a consultant to the films "Greystoke" and "Project X," and the television program "Quantum Leap."

Stephen R. Kaufman, M.D.

Dr. Kaufman is a Clinical Instructor at Case Western Reserve University. He received a B.A. from Yale University and an M.D. from Case Western Reserve University. He completed an ophthalmology residency at New York University Medical Center and a retina fellowship at Manhattan Eye Ear & Throat Hospital. He is certified by the American Board of Ophthalmology. He has published articles on macular diseases and laser therapy. He was the principal investigator of a review of animal models of human diseases, published as Volume 1 supplement of *Perspectives on Animal Research*. He is the Co-Chair of the Medical Research Modernization Committee, co-editor of *Perspectives on Medical Research*, and Vice-President of the Center for Health Research Policy.

Marvin F. Kraushar, M.D.

Dr. Kraushar is a Clinical Professor of Ophthalmology at the University of Medicine and Dentistry of New Jersey and an Associate Clinical Professor of Ophthalmology at the Mount Sinai School of Medicine. He received his A.B. from Bowdoin College and M.D. from Tufts University School of Medicine. He did an ophthalmology residency at Brooklyn Eye & Ear Hospital and a fellowship in retinal detachment at the Massachusetts Eye & Ear Infirmary. He is certified by the American Board of Ophthalmology and the American Board of Laser Surgery. He has published 47 papers and presented 207 papers by invitation.

Deanna Z. Macek, M.D.

Dr. Macek was an Assistant Clinical Professor of Ophthalmology at the New York Medical College from 1979-1990, and she is currently in private practice. She majored in biology at The State College, Beroun, Czechoslovakia and did medical training at The Charles' University School of Medicine in Pilsen, Czechoslovakia. She did ophthalmology residency training at Hahnemann Medical College and a fellowship in fluorescein angiography and retinal vascular disorders at Johns Hopkins Hospital. She has published in the area of fluorescein angiography, and she is certified by the American Board of Ophthalmology.

Brandon P. Reines, D.V.M.

Dr. Reines received his B.S. from the University of Massachusetts and D.V.M. from Tufts University. He is President of The Center for Health Science Policy in Washington, DC. He has published articles on medical discovery in *Perspectives in Biology and Medicine* and *The Journal of Medicine and Philosophy*. His monographs include *Cancer Research on Animals: Impact and Alternatives, Heart Research on Animals: A Critique of Animal Models of Cardiovascular Disease, Psychology Experiments on Animals: A Critique of Animal Models of Human Psychopathology,* and *Environmental Experiments on Animals: A Critique of Animal Models of Heatstroke, Frostbite, and Hypoxemia.*

Increased Understanding of Sickle-Cell Anemia: A Result of Clinical and *In Vitro* Research

Eric Dunayer

Sickle-cell anemia (SCA) is an inherited disorder caused by abnormal hemoglobin. In humans, normal adult hemoglobin consists of two pairs of globular proteins, with each pair composed of an α-globin chain and a β-globin chain.[1] In most cases of SCA, a single mutation causes the amino acid valine, located at a particular point in hemoglobin's β-globin chains, to be replaced by another amino acid, glutamine.[2] As a result, the body's hemoglobin becomes unstable under low-oxygen conditions: individual hemoglobin molecules deform, becoming insoluble and gelatinous. When enough hemoglobin in a particular red blood cell gels, the cell changes shape; instead of resembling a disk centrally concave on both sides, as is normal, the cell now resembles a sickle.[1]

Unlike normal red blood cells, sickled cells cannot bend in order to pass through narrow blood passageways. Because the spleen's blood passageways are particularly narrow, sickled red blood cells are especially likely to lodge in the spleen, which destroys them; when a sufficient number are destroyed, the result is anemia. In addition, sickled cells often adhere to blood vessels, causing them to become blocked. Such vaso-occlusion leads to severe pain, cumulative organ dysfunction, and eventually death.[1]

The sickle-cell gene is inherited as an autosomal dominant. Those heterozygous for the gene carry the sickle-cell trait. Such "carriers" show no signs of the disease unless exposed to conditions of extremely low oxygen--for example, at high altitudes. In the United States approximately 8% of blacks carry the sickle-cell trait. Individuals homozygous for the sickle-cell gene nearly always suffer from SCA. Approximately 0.2% (1 in 500) of American blacks are homozygous for this gene.[3]

Currently no effective SCA therapy exists. Treatment is merely palliative, aimed at relieving pain during vaso-occlusive crises and reducing organ damage.[4]

Information about sickle-cell trait and SCA has come almost exclusively from human clinical studies and *in vitro* studies of human-derived cells or molecules.

Until recently no animal "models" mimicked SCA's spontaneous sickling of red blood cells or the long-term effects of SCA's vaso-occlusive events.[4] In an effort to find an adequate animal model of SCA, researchers have now inserted human genes that code for sickle-cell hemoglobin into mouse embryos.[4-9] In some cases the resulting transgenic mice have shown symptoms resembling those commonly seen in SCA; the mice's symptoms, however, are milder.[4-9] To date, research with transgenic mice has failed to advance our understanding or treatment of SCA.

Fetal Hemoglobin's Capacity to Inhibit Sickling: Insights from Clinical and *In Vitro* Studies

Most SCA research seeks to increase production of fetal hemoglobin, which has anti-sickling properties. These properties were uncovered by human clinical studies involving *in vitro* methods.

In humans, red blood cells normally produce fetal hemoglobin (composed of α-globin and γ-globin chains) *in utero* until about 30 weeks of gestation. Hemoglobin production then almost entirely switches to production of adult hemoglobin (α-globin and β-globin chains).[10] However, red blood cells containing fetal hemoglobin continue to circulate for some time after an infant's birth. Normally a newborn's blood is about 80% fetal hemoglobin; by the time the infant is 4½ months old, adult hemoglobin has largely replaced fetal hemoglobin, which few cells then contain.[11]

In 1948 pediatrician Janet Watson tested 226 black mothers and their newborns for sickled red blood cells. Eight percent of the mothers and 8.4% of the infants tested positive, showing red blood cells that sickled *in vitro* under low-oxygen conditions. The *percentage* of red cells that sickled *in vitro*, however, differed sharply between the two "positive" groups: in the mothers it was nearly 100%, but in the infants it averaged only 11% (ranging from 0.5% to 30%).[11] Watson then hypothesized that fetal hemoglobin might inhibit sickling--in which case the rate of sickling should increase as adult hemoglobin replaces fetal hemoglobin. To continue study on infants who showed sickling, Watson followed 11 of them to four months of age, by which time over 90% of each infant's red blood cells sickled *in vitro*.[11] In further support of Watson's theory, other researchers soon found that, among adults with SCA, those few with at least 20% fetal hemoglobin have milder clinical symptoms.[12,13]

After researchers had demonstrated that fetal hemoglobin inhibits sickling and lessens SCA's severity, hematologist Thalia Papayannopoulou and colleagues examined whether or not it was possible to increase the number of red blood cells producing fetal hemoglobin in adult humans. In 1976 Papayannopoulou's research group cultured bone-marrow cells from adult humans and found that as the number of red blood cells increased so did the number of cells producing fetal hemoglobin. Consequently they hypothesized that it might be possible to reactivate fetal-hemoglobin production in adults.[14]

Screening for Drugs to Increase Fetal Hemoglobin: The Futile Use of Baboons

However, research on fetal hemoglobin soon became increasingly animal-oriented--after Joseph DeSimone and colleagues discovered in 1978 that baboons, like humans, normally show a progression from fetal to adult hemoglobin production.[15,16]

Because Papayannopoulou et al.'s work with human bone-marrow culture had suggested that an increase in red blood cell production can be accompanied by an increase in fetal-hemoglobin production, DeSimone and colleagues next hypothesized that it might be possible to increase fetal-hemoglobin production in baboons by increasing *their* red blood cell production.[16] Since anemia induced by particular drugs or by blood loss ordinarily leads to a compensatory increase in red blood cell production, DeSimone's group artificially induced anemia in baboons with drugs and/or bloodletting.[15,16] One group of baboons responded by producing 10% of their replacement hemoglobin as fetal hemoglobin; these baboons were designated "high responders." Those baboons who produced less than 2% fetal hemoglobin were designated "low responders."[15]

DeSimone et al. then explored using baboons to screen for drugs capable of increasing fetal-hemoglobin production.[16] The first drug to be tested, 5-Azacytidine (5-AZA), was known to counter normal biochemical inhibition of the expression of some genes, including the gene for fetal hemoglobin.[1] In 1982 DeSimone and colleagues bled two groups of high-responder baboons to induce anemia; they then administered 5-AZA to one of the groups. On average about 60% of the replacement hemoglobin produced by the baboons who had received 5-AZA was fetal hemoglobin; in contrast, the control-group baboons produced only about 10% fetal hemoglobin.[15]

When, in 1983, 5-AZA was tried in SCA patients, preliminary results were not nearly as promising as in high-responder baboons: in the patients 5-AZA generally increased fetal-hemoglobin levels to only 6-18%.[1,17] Epidemiological studies of SCA patients with naturally occurring fetal hemoglobin had previously shown that the percentage of fetal hemoglobin must be 20-40% to be therapeutic.[17] In any case, human trials of 5-AZA were soon abandoned, after researchers found that the drug causes carcinomas in rats.[16]

Hematologist Adil Al-Khatti and colleagues soon tested another potential anti-sickling drug on anemic high-responder baboons--recombinant erythropoietin, a genetically engineered form of a naturally occurring hormone that regulates production of red blood cells. In 1987 they reported that erythropoietin increased the percentage of fetal hemoglobin from approximately 10% to as high as 50%.[18] However, a decade earlier Papayannopoulou et al. had already shown, in human bone-marrow culture, that erythropoietin increases the percentage of cells containing fetal hemoglobin.[1,19] In addition, when Al-Khatti et al. conducted their baboon research on erythropoietin, the hormone was already being used to treat the anemia that often accompanies kidney failure in humans. The hypothesis that erythropoietin increases fetal-hemoglobin production could easily have been tested clinically, in patients with anemia related to kidney failure or with SCA.[18] When in 1991 erythropoietin was finally clinically tested in humans with SCA, it did *not* dramatically increase fetal-hemoglobin production, as it had in the baboon subjects.[1] The baboons used in fetal-hemoglobin research cannot serve to predict the magnitude of humans' fetal-hemoglobin response to drugs.

More generally, baboons and humans show species differences that preclude the validity of SCA work in baboons. For example, the two species differ in the way fetal hemoglobin is distributed among their red blood cells. In baboons fetal hemoglobin tends to be evenly distributed among all red blood cells; in humans it tends to appear only in a small percentage of cells.[19] Therefore, drugs intended to increase fetal-hemoglobin production in humans can increase it only in proportionately few cells. Since only these cells might then resist sickling, the problems associated with sickling would continue.[17]

Clearly the use of baboons is an ineffective way of seeking information on fetal-hemoglobin production in humans.

Butyrates' Capacity to Increase Fetal Hemoglobin: Another Discovery from Clinical and *In Vitro* Research

Insights into another potential way of increasing fetal-hemoglobin production have also derived exclusively from clinical and *in vitro* research.

Diabetics experience bouts of abnormally high blood-glucose levels. During the pregnancy of a diabetic woman, excess glucose periodically crosses the placenta; the fetus responds by producing more insulin, which reduces glucose levels.[10] Because insulin has been shown to affect gene expression, in the 1980s Susan Perrine and colleagues examined red blood cells from newborns of diabetic mothers to see whether insulin affected expression of the gene for fetal hemoglobin. The group found that the newborns did show a delayed switch from fetal to adult hemoglobin production.[10] Using cultured blood cells from the umbilical cords of newborns whose mothers were *not* diabetic, Perrine et al. then tested various substances known to be elevated in diabetes. They found that some butyrates (fatty acids) increase fetal-hemoglobin production.[20]

Next the researchers infused sheep fetuses--*in utero*--with butyrates. The fetuses showed a delayed switch from fetal to adult hemoglobin.[21] Providing no new insights, this finding simply paralleled the prior clinical and *in vitro* findings.

The therapeutic implications of butyrates' effect on hemoglobin production have yet to be demonstrated.

Unsuccessful Efforts to Contrive an Adequate Animal Model of SCA

In various nonhuman animals--including deer, goats, hamsters, mongooses, raccoons, sheep, and squirrels--red blood cells sometimes naturally sickle.[22] However, as pathologists Robert Nalbandian and colleagues note in a letter to *The New England Journal of Medicine*, the sickling that occurs in these animals' red blood cells is generally independent of oxygen concentration, may be reversed by changes in pH, and occurs (*in vitro*) in high-concentration salt solutions or after prolonged storage of cells. Sickling of *human* cells shows none of these characteristics. Nalbandian et al. conclude, "The mechanisms involved and very probably the molecular pathology in these animal models differ considerably from that postulated [for SCA]."[22]

Because the naturally occurring mutation that causes SCA is apparently unique to humans, in 1988 Edward Rubin et al. inserted the human gene that codes for sickle-cell hemoglobin into mouse embryos, in the hope that the red blood cells of the resulting transgenic mice would then sickle.[4] Unlike humans, mice normally have two types of β-globin in their red blood cells--major and minor.[4] Since in humans normal β-globin inhibits sickling, the researchers used a strain of mice who suffer from β-thalassemia, a condition in which major β-globin is absent. Some of the resulting transgenic mice produced sickle-cell hemoglobin and passed the gene for such hemoglobin on to their offspring. In no mouse, however, did any red blood cells sickle.[4] (The mice's minor β-globin may have prevented sickling.)[4]

In 1990 David Greaves and colleagues also inserted the SCA gene into mouse embryos. Because in humans sickle-cell hemoglobin is composed of α-globin and abnormal β-globin chains, the researchers inserted genes, joined together, for both of these globin chains. Three of the five transgenic mice born showed sickle-cell hemoglobin, comprising 10%, 35%, and 83% of their total hemoglobin. These three mice also produced red blood cells that sickled *in vitro*. However, as revealed by blood smears, two of the three mice with blood cells that sickled *in vitro* showed no *in vivo* sickling.[5] Further, whereas in humans with SCA the percentage of sickled cells *in vivo* is 6-32%,[23] in the transgenic mouse who showed *in vivo* sickling the percentage was only about 0.1%. None of the mice had any SCA-like symptoms, including anemia.[5] The mice were then crossbred with β-thalassemic mice. The resulting offspring had over 90% sickled cells *in vitro*. Although these mice showed anemia and enlarged spleens, the symptoms were milder than in most SCA and the mice were otherwise healthy.[6]

Since implanting the human gene for the most common form of sickle-cell hemoglobin did not cause SCA in mice, researchers turned to two less common forms (S-Antilles and D Punjab) that contain two abnormal amino acids (rather than one) and so cause disease even in humans heterozygous for the sickle-cell gene. In 1991, Marie Trudel et al. reported joining S-Antilles and D Punjab hemoglobin genes and inserting them into mouse embryos. As the researchers had desired, the resulting transgenic mice produced sickle-cell hemoglobin, which the researchers dubbed "hemoglobin SAD" (for **S**-**A**ntilles/**D** Punjab).[7] When these mice were bred with normal mice, the offspring produced approximately 20% of their hemoglobin as hemoglobin SAD. The offspring also had slightly enlarged spleens and some sickled red blood cells but were not anemic.[7] When the first-generation transgenic mice were bred with β-thalassemic mice, the offspring had approximately 26% hemoglobin SAD as well as more sickled cells *in vivo* and more destruction of red blood cells than the mice with 20% hemoglobin SAD. Exposed to conditions of very low oxygen (atmospheric concentration of only 8% as opposed to the normal 21%), these mice died, possibly from vaso-occlusion caused by severe sickling.[7]

Although hemoglobin-SAD mice possess red blood cells that sickle *in vivo*, particularly under conditions of very low oxygen, there are serious scientific problems with using these mice to investigate SCA.

First, unlike most sickle-cell hemoglobin, hemoglobin SAD has *two* abnormal amino acids rather than one; arising from a different mutation, it has a different molecular basis for its instability.[7] Researchers have claimed that hemoglobin-SAD mice can be useful in the search for drugs to reduce or prevent sickling,[4] but agents that stabilize hemoglobin SAD may not stabilize the more common sickle-cell hemoglobin, and vice versa.

More importantly, species differences render the use of mice for SCA research fundamentally unsound. Unlike humans, mice have no distinct fetal hemoglobin: until 11 days of gestation, fetal mice produce three β-like globins that closely resemble adult mouse hemoglobin; for the remainder of gestation, they produce adult hemoglobin.[8] Further, in humans the switch from fetal to adult hemoglobin is reversible, whereas in mice the switch from the three initial β-like globins to two adult β-globins is apparently irreversible.[8] Therefore, possible methods of reactivating fetal hemoglobin--the focus of most SCA research--cannot be tested in mice. Also, human SCA patients often suffer kidney damage, even kidney failure, from a succession of vaso-occlusive episodes; in the mouse kidney, blood vessels are proportionately wider and therefore at less risk of becoming obstructed.[9] As hematologist Mary Fabray and colleagues conclude, "The transgenic mouse (as any other animal model) will necessarily differ substantially from the sickle cell disease patient because mouse anatomy and physiology differ from human."[9]

Conclusion

Advances in understanding SCA have come almost exclusively from human clinical research and *in vitro* studies of human-derived cells or molecules. Although animal "models" have been used in efforts to discover ways of preventing or countering the sickling of red blood cells, fundamental species differences have undermined such efforts. These differences will, almost certainly, continue to prevent animal experimentation from making any significant contribution to the prevention or treatment of SCA.

References

1. Stamatoyannopoulos JA, Nienhuis AW: Therapeutic approaches to hemoglobin switching in treatment of hemoglobinopathies. *Ann Rev of Med* 1992;43:497-521.
2. Nagel RL: Severity, pathobiology, epistatic effects, and genetic markers in sickle cell anemia. *Sem in Hematol* 1991;28:180-201.
3. Steinberg MH: Review: The sickle hemoglobinopathies--genetic analysis of common phenocopies and new molecular approaches to treatment. *Am J Med Sci* 1984;288:169-174.
4. Rubin EM, Lu R, Cooper S, Mohandas N, Kan YW: Introduction and expression of the human B^s-globin gene in transgenic mice. *Am J Hum Genetics* 1988;42:585-591.
5. Greaves DR, Fraser P, Vidal MA, Hedges MJ, Ropers D, Luzzatto L, Grosveld F: A transgenic mouse model of sickle cell disorder. *Nature* 1990;343:183-185.
6. Ryan TM, Townes TM, Reilly MP, Asakura T, Palmiter RD, Brinster RL, Behringer RR: Human sickle hemoglobin in transgenic mice. *Science* 1990;247:566-568.
7. Trudel M, Saadane N, Garel M-C, Bardakdijian-Michau J, Blouquit Y, Guerquin-Kern J-L, Rouyer-Fessard P, Vidaud D, Pachnis A, Roméo P-H, Bouzard Y, Constantini F: Towards a transgenic mouse model of sickle cell disease: Hemoglobin SAD. *The EMBO J* 1991;10:3157-3165.
8. Albitar M, Makoto K, Liebhaber SA: Human α-globin genes demonstrate autonomous developmental regulation in transgenic mice. *Mol and Cell Biol* 1991;11:3786-3794.
9. Fabray ME, Constantini F, Pachnis A, Suzuka SM, Bank N, Aynedjian HS, Factor SM, Nagel RL: High expression of human β^S- and α-globins in transgenic mice: Erythrocyte abnormalities, organ damage, and effect of hypoxia. *Proc Natl Acad Sci USA* 1992;89:12155-12159.
10. Perrine SP, Greene MF, Faller DV: Delay in the fetal globin switch in infants of diabetic mothers. *NEJM* 1985;312:334-338.
11. Watson J: The significance of the paucity of sickle cells in newborn negro infants. *Am J Med Sci* 1948;215:419-423.
12. Herman EC, Jr., Conley CL: Hereditary persistence of fetal hemoglobin: A family study. *Am J Med* 1960;29:9-17.
13. Dover GJ, Charache S: Chemotherapy and hemoglobin F synthesis in sickle cell disease. *Ann NY Acad Sci* 1989;565:222-227.
14. Papayannopoulou T, Brice M, Stamatoyannopoulos G: Stimulation of fetal hemoglobin synthesis in bone marrow cultures from adult individuals. *Proc Natl Acad Sci USA* 1976;73:2033-2037.
15. DeSimone J, Heller P, Hall L, Zwiers D: 5-Azacytidine stimulates fetal hemoglobin synthesis in anemic baboons. *Proc Natl Acad Sci USA* 1982;79:4428-4431.
16. Heller P, DeSimone J: 5-Azacytidine and fetal hemoglobin. *Amer J Hematol* 1984;17: 439-447.
17. Noguchi CT, Rodgers GP, Serjeant G, Schechter AN: Levels of fetal hemoglobin

necessary for treatment of sickle cell disease. *NEJM* 1988;318:96-99.

18. Al-Khatti A, Veith RW, Papayannopoulou T, Fritsch EF, Goldwasser E, Stamatoyannopoulos G: Stimulation of fetal hemoglobin synthesis by erythropoietin in baboons. *NEJM* 1987;317:415-420.
19. Lavelle D, DeSimone J, Heller P: Fetal hemoglobin reactivation in baboon and man: A short perspective. *Amer J Hematol* 1993;42:91-95.
20. Perrine SP, Miller BA, Greene MF, Cohen RF, Cook N, Shackleton C, Faller DV: Butyric acid analogues augment γ globin gene expression in neonatal erythroid progenitors. *Biochem and Biophys Res Comm* 1987;148:694-700.
21. Perrine SP, Swerdlow P, Faller DV, Qin G, Rudolph AM, Reczek J, Kan YW: Butyric acid modulates developmental globin gene switching in man and sheep. *Adv Exp Mol Biol* 1989;271:177-183.
22. Nalbandian RM, Kessler DL, Henry R: Anthropoid diseases in animals (letter). *NEJM* 1970;282:103-104.
23. Castro O, Roth R, Orlin J, Finch SC: Human sickle cells in a heterologous species: A model for the screening of anti-sickling agents, in Brewer GJ (ed): *Erythrocyte Structure and Function* New York, Alan R. Liss, Inc, 1975.

The Failure of Animal Models of Cystic Fibrosis

Eric Dunayer

Introduction: The Human Disease

Cystic fibrosis (CF) is a progressive disease characterized by dysfunction of the secretory epithelial cells that line the sweat glands, salivary glands, intestines, pancreas, trachea, and bronchi.[1] CF's pulmonary manifestations--thickened mucus that is difficult to expectorate, recurrent bacterial infection, and destruction of lung tissue--account for most symptoms and deaths caused by the disease. Ultimately CF is fatal.[2]

Inherited as a recessive trait, CF is one of the commonest human genetic diseases, affecting about one in 2,000 children. In the United States, eight million (one in 31) people are believed to carry a CF gene.[1]

CF arises from a defect in the gene that codes for the protein "cystic fibrosis transmembrane regulator" (CFTR).[3] While some of its functions have yet to be elucidated, CFTR is believed to span the width of a cell's membrane and act as a channel through which chloride ions pass into and out of the cell. (Alternatively, CFTR may indirectly control the passage of chloride ions by activating *another* protein that serves as the chloride-ion channel.) In CF patients, the CFTR present in certain types of secretory epithelial cells fails to respond to biochemical cues that these cells should either absorb or secrete chloride ions; instead the chloride-ion channels remain closed.[1,4] Defective chloride-ion transport leads to CF's symptoms.[2]

In normal individuals, chloride ions transported into the trachea and bronchi draw water into these airways; the water hydrates secretions and keeps them fluid. Because CF patients lack this chloride-ion transport, their respiratory secretions become thickened and difficult to expectorate. The thickened mucus provides a site for chronic bacterial infection. White blood cells, drawn to the lungs by this infection, degenerate and add their DNA to the already-thickened mixture, further increasing viscosity. Eventually airway obstruction impairs respiration, leads to the destruction of lung tissue, and proves fatal.[2]

Advances in understanding and treating CF have derived from clinical and *in vitro* research. CF researchers (including a number of animal experimenters) generally agree that there is no valid animal "model" of CF.[5-8] Nevertheless, researchers continue to propose various animal models, either naturally occurring (genetic) or artificially induced.

Clinical and *In Vitro* Advances

Improved diagnosis and supportive care, as well as an increased emphasis on therapies that focus on CF's respiratory symptoms, have extended the life expectancy of CF patients--from the pre-teens in the 1940s to the mid- to late-twenties today.[1] Antibiotics have proved beneficial in controlling CF-associated bacterial lung infections.[1] Various other drugs, such as deoxyribonuclease (DNase) and acetylcysteine, have been partially effective in thinning CF's tenacious respiratory secretions and facilitating their clearance; these drugs are administered as aerosols.[1]

The use of aerosolized drugs to loosen pulmonary secretions followed a serendipitous observation in tuberculosis patients. In the 1940s, clinicians such as Joseph B. Miller were treating tuberculosis by administering the antibiotic streptomycin in an aerosol inhalant containing the detergent Triton A-20. These clinicians noted that Triton A-20 had a side-effect of liquefying sputum. Before treatment, the patients had difficulty clearing bronchial secretions. "Almost immediately after beginning treatment with Triton A-20 aerosols," Miller recalls, "their secretions became thin and watery" and were easily expectorated. Triton A-20 was then used to treat other chronic pulmonary diseases, including CF. The "thinning effect was found to be constant and dependable," Miller notes.[9] (After Triton A-20 had been widely and safely used in children and adults for years, Miller and Edward H. Boyer conducted Triton A-20 toxicity tests in rats. Their finding of no pulmonary toxicity was "in complete agreement with the clinical experiences"--and apparently superfluous.)[9]

Following Triton A-20's success, researchers sought other drugs that liquefy respiratory secretions. To better identify agents capable of thinning these secretions, investigators collected sputum from CF patients and analyzed its composition. CF bronchial secretions, they found, have considerably higher DNA concentration than bronchial secretions resulting from other pulmonary diseases.[10,11] In CF, as previously mentioned, white blood cells drawn to the lungs by infection degenerate, releasing DNA that forms a gel and mixes with already-thickened mucus to further increase sputum viscosity.[2,10,11] By mixing sputum samples from CF patients with various agents, researchers screened for drugs that decrease the viscosity of CF secretions. *In vitro*, bovine pancreatic DNase I (an enzyme that digests DNA) was found to be especially effective.[12,13] Clinical trials showed that bovine DNase was effective in treating CF; in 1958 it was approved for use.[13] In following years, however, clinicians noted occasional adverse respiratory reactions--perhaps allergic reactions to bovine protein in the enzyme, perhaps reactions to cell damage caused by contaminants (other bovine pancreatic enzymes) in the DNase solution.[13] Recently a recombinant human DNase (rhDNase) produced in human embryonic kidney cells was evaluated *in vitro* using sputum from CF patients; the rhDNase rapidly thinned the sputum.[13] A preliminary study of rhDNase in CF patients has indicated that the enzyme is safe and effective in thinning respiratory secretions.[2]

Like the finding of high DNA levels in CF secretions, the link between CF and defective ion transport was first discovered in CF patients. During a 1948 heat wave in New York City, clinicians W. R. Kessler and Dorothy H. Andersen noted that 5 out of 10 children admitted to Babies Hospital for heat prostration had previously been diagnosed with CF. In a 1951 *Pediatrics* paper, they speculated that children with CF might be especially prone to heat prostration.[14] Based on this report, pediatrician Paul A. di Sant'Agnese and his colleagues exposed normal children and those with CF to an ambient temperature of 90°F and collected their sweat for study. In the sweat of CF patients, chloride-ion concentrations were triple those of normal controls; sodium-ion levels, too, were greatly elevated. Urine analysis revealed that in CF patients the kidneys conserve chloride and sodium ions, but continued and uncontrolled loss of these ions through sweat eventually leads to heat prostration.[15] These findings confirmed clinical impressions that CF patients are particularly vulnerable to heat stress and indicated that CF affects more of the body's physiology than had previously been realized; they also strongly supported the hypothesis that CF involves a defect in ion transport.[15]

The precise nature of CF's ion-transport defect was determined *in vitro*. In the 1980s, Paul Quinton demonstrated that chloride ions cannot penetrate the membranes of certain types of cells from CF patients.[1] The major breakthrough in understanding CF's molecular basis came in 1989 when, using *in vitro* techniques, researchers studying human molecular genetics pinpointed a defective gene (the CFTR gene) in CF patients that they suspected was responsible for causing the disease.[1] Within a year, researchers transferred a normal human CFTR gene, *in vitro*, into airway[4] and pancreatic[16] epithelial cells from CF patients; the cells acquired the ability to transport chloride ions normally. This *in vitro* work confirmed that a mutant CFTR gene causes CF's defect in chloride-ion transport and indicated that transfer of a normal CFTR gene might normalize chloride-ion transport in CF patients.[4,16]

Transfer of the Normal Human CFTR Gene to Rats

In work reported in 1992, Melissa A. Rosenfeld et al. transferred a normal human CFTR gene--*in vitro*--into epithelial cells from CF patients by infecting these cells with Ad-CFTR, replication-deficient adenovirus containing the CFTR gene. The cells then produced structurally normal human CFTR and showed normal chloride-ion transport.[8]

Rosenfeld and her colleagues *followed* this *in vitro* success with an *in vivo* demonstration. Again using Ad-CFTR infection, they transferred a normal human CFTR gene into epithelial cells in the lungs of cotton rats. Like the cells from CF patients, the cells in the rats' lungs responded to the transfer by producing structurally normal human CFTR. With regard to this result of gene transfer, then, the rat work merely duplicated previous *in vitro* work. The rat work was even less useful with regard to the transfer's effect on chloride-ion transport: Unlike the *in vitro* research, the rat research could not reveal whether transfer of a normal human CFTR gene can correct a defect in chloride-ion transport--because the rats never had such a defect. Rosenfeld et al. acknowledge, "As there is no animal model for cystic fibrosis, it is not possible to demonstrate definitively the function of the Ad-CFTR-directed CFTR protein *in vivo*."[8]

To date, progress in transfer of the normal human CFTR gene has derived from *in vitro* work, not animal experimentation.

Animal Models of CF

Two genetic diseases in mice have been studied as models of CF. One of these diseases, a "cribriform degeneration" suffered by some DBA/2J mice, involves degeneration of the central nervous system characterized by cell death that leaves scattered cavities in the brain and spinal cord. At about 2½ to 3 weeks of age, mice with cribriform degeneration begin to show stunted growth, overall weakness, and incoordination.[17] Because the sweat of CF patients had shown elevated levels of sodium and chloride ions,[15] the finding, in the early 1970s, that mice with cribriform degeneration have abnormally high sodium-ion levels in their fur sparked interest in this disease as a model of CF.[17] However, researchers soon discovered that the abnormally high sodium-ion concentrations in the fur of the mice is *not* accompanied by sweat-gland dysfunction (which occurs in CF). The only ion-transport dysfunction found was excessive sodium-ion secretion by the parotid salivary glands. Through their saliva, the mice were transferring sodium ions to their fur--by licking themselves during grooming.[17] In addition, the researchers' focus on sodium ions would later prove to have been misguided: Paul Quinton's *in vitro* work would reveal that CF arises from a defect in the transport of chloride, not sodium, ions.[1]

Another proposed genetic model of CF involves the use of CBA/J mice. Like CF patients, some CBA/J mice suffer from exocrine pancreatic insufficiency (EPI), inadequate secretion of digestive enzymes produced in the pancreas. For this reason, mouse EPI has been suggested as a model of the EPI of CF patients.[18] Although both EPIs result from the destruction of pancreatic cells, the causes of the cell destruction fundamentally differ.[19-21] In CF patients, the destruction results from obstruction of the pancreatic ducts by thickened secretions;[19] in CBA/J mice, it results from digestive enzymes produced in the pancreas being activated within the pancreatic cells themselves (instead of being secreted into the small intestine and activated there, as is normal).[20,21] Because mouse EPI and the EPI of CF patients have different causes, the mouse model is unlikely to reveal ways of halting the pancreatic destruction that accompanies CF.

Other researchers have used artificially induced bacterial infection in nonhuman animals as a model of the pulmonary infection seen in CF patients.[5] For decades, it has been known that the vast majority of teenage CF patients suffer recurrent respiratory infection by the bacterium *Pseudomonas aeruginosa*--infection associated with increased morbidity and mortality.[5] Among those who do *not* suffer this chronic infection, many have developed opsonizing antibodies (antibodies that facilitate white blood cells' engulfment and destruction of bacteria) against mucoid exopolysaccharide (MEP), a carbohydrate in the bacterium's outer coat.[5] Following clinical observation of the benefits of opsonizing MEP antibodies, experimenters examined whether these antibodies confer protection against *P. aeruginosa* in nonhuman animals as well. Gerald B. Pier and colleagues injected rats and mice with MEP and then exposed them, via the trachea, to *P. aeruginosa*. Those animals who had responded to MEP injection by producing opsonizing MEP antibodies developed significantly fewer *P. aeruginosa* infections than those who had not produced these antibodies. These findings, however, provided no new information of any practical significance; they merely paralleled findings in CF patients.[5]

The most popular CF animal models involve the use of drugs to impair the autonomic nervous system (ANS), which regulates involuntary functions. Drugs such as isoproterenol or pilocarpine are sometimes used to block the action of catecholamines (neurotransmitters active in the ANS) and create symptoms similar to those seen in CF. Usually, however, reserpine is used to deplete catecholamine reserves and thereby impair the ANS.[22]

In the mid-1970s, researchers introduced reserpine-induced ANS dysfunction as a model of CF.[18] In rats, seven daily reserpine injections cause an accumulation of secretions that blocks the ducts of some exocrine glands.[22,23] This blockage resembles that in CF.[22] Although reserpine-treated rats produce excessive intestinal mucus,[22,23] as do CF patients,[23] the rat mucus differs from the human mucus in biochemical composition.[23] In addition, the cause of exocrine-gland pathology in CF (a defect in chloride-ion transport)[1] fundamentally differs from the cause in reserpine-treated rats (ANS dysfunction).[18,22] Originally the reserpine-treated rat (RR) model arose from the belief that faulty ANS control caused the dysfunction of some exocrine glands in CF.[18] Since then, however, *in vitro* work has shown that CF exocrine-gland pathology is due to an inherent molecular flaw in the secretory epithelial cells of exocrine glands, not to abnormal ANS innervation.[22]

Studies of the RR model of CF have continued because reserpine-treated rats possess some secretory epithelial cells (for example, in the pancreas, salivary glands, and trachea) that appear to have a chloride-ion transport defect.[24] Researchers have found, however, that ion transport in rats treated with reserpine or other compounds that impair the ANS differs in important ways from ion transport in CF patients. In the 1980s, human studies revealed that in CF patients the epithelial cells of the nose, trachea, and bronchi have an electrical potential difference, or PD (the difference in charge between a cell's inside and outside) of approximately -50 mV, while in control subjects the PD is approximately -20 mV.[6] The PD is more negative in CF patients because their respiratory epithelial cells can absorb sodium ions (which are positively charged) but not chloride ions (negatively charged)--creating excess negativity outside the cell. Following these clinical findings, Duncan F. Rogers et al. treated rats with reserpine and isoproterenol and measured the effects on the PD of tracheal epithelial cells *in vivo*. The treatments did not produce the desired increase in PD negativity; instead, the tracheal PD of the treated rats did not significantly differ from that of controls. Rogers et al. concluded that the imbalance in ion absorption that produces excessively negative airway PD in CF patients is, in all likelihood, "not present in these models."[6]

As reported by gastroenterologist H. J. Veeze and colleagues, CF and the RR model also appear to differ in intestinal chloride-ion transport: In CF patients this transport is blocked, but in reserpine-treated rats it is normal. Veeze et al. conducted *in vitro* work in which they treated cells from the small intestine of CF patients with various drugs and metabolites that stimulate chloride-ion secretion in normal human intestinal cells. As expected, the treated cells failed to secrete chloride ions. In contrast, when Veeze et al. exposed cells from the large intestine of reserpine-treated rats to these same compounds, the cells did secrete chloride ions. The researchers interpreted the results as indicating "normal function and regulation" of intestinal chloride-ion channels in the reserpine-treated rat.[25]

Further, in humans, CFTR-mediated chloride-ion transport (defective in CF patients) is regulated primarily by the metabolite cyclic AMP, with a minor contribution from calcium ions.[24] In rats, however, calcium ions are the major regulator of chloride-ion transport--at least in the pancreas and salivary glands, where chloride-ion transport is impaired by reserpine.[24] Because of these differences, J. Ricardo Martinez and A. M. Martinez have written that studies of pancreatic and salivary cells in reserpine-treated rats are of questionable relevance to CF.[24]

Most recently, animal experimenters have attempted to study CF by means of a transgenic-mouse model. In 1992 J.N. Snouwaert and colleagues announced that they had produced transgenic mice who carry a defective human CFTR gene and, as a consequence, lack functional CFTR.[26] Although researchers working with the transgenic-mouse model are touting it as a breakthrough,[26-28] the pathology in the transgenic mice significantly differs from that in CF. In the mice, the primary pathology is intestinal obstruction due to thickened mucus. Most CF patients, however, do not experience intestinal obstruction.[26] Further, the mice do not manifest the pancreatic, reproductive, or respiratory pathologies found in CF.[26,27] Although they show abnormal chloride transport in nasal epithelial cells and some increase in the number of tracheal cells that produce mucus, the mice do not develop pulmonary obstructive disease--the most life-threatening feature of CF.[26,27] A number of factors could underlie the absence of pulmonary obstruction in the mice. Compared to humans, mice have far fewer mucus-producing glands lining their trachea.[27] Also, unlike humans, mice possess a second ion-transport system in their airway; this second system may compensate, at least partially, for the loss of functional CFTR.[27,28] Given these major differences in pathology, anatomy, and physiology between humans and mice, how can data obtained from the transgenic mice be meaningfully extrapolated to humans? The transgenic-mouse model is highly unlikely to provide insights applicable to treatment of CF.

Conclusion

The history of cystic fibrosis research reveals that progress in understanding and treating the disease has derived from clinical and *in vitro* studies. Researchers generally agree that no valid animal model of cystic fibrosis exists. The animal models currently being manipulated or proposed are fundamentally flawed.

References

1. Davies K. Cystic fibrosis: The quest for a cure. *New Scientist* 7 December 1991:30-34.
2. Hubbard RC, McElvaney NG, Birrer P, Shak S, Robinson WW, Jolley C, Wu M, Chernick MS, Crystal RG. A preliminary study of aerosolized recombinant human deoxyribonuclease I in the treatment of cystic fibrosis. *N Eng J Med* 1992;326:812-815.
3. Tata F, Stanier P, Wicking C, Halford S, Kruyer H, Lench NJ, Scambler PJ, Hansen C, Branman JC, Williamson R, Wainwright BJ. Cloning the mouse homolog of the human cystic fibrosis transmembrane conductance regulator gene. *Genomics* 1991;10: 301-307.
4. Rich DP, Anderson MP, Gregory RJ, Cheng SH, Paul S, Jefferson DM, McCann JD, Klinger KW, Smith AE, Welsh MJ. Expression of cystic fibrosis transmembrane conductance regulator corrects defective chloride channel regulation in cystic fibrosis airway epithelial cells. *Nature* 1990;347:358-363.
5. Pier GB, Small GJ, Warren HB. Protection against mucoid *Pseudomonas aeruginosa* in rodent models of endobronchial infection. *Science* 1990;249:537-540.
6. Rogers DF, Alton EW, Dewar A, Geddes DM, Barnes PJ. Tracheal potential difference in the reserpine and isoproterenol rat models of cystic fibrosis. *Exp Lung Res* 1990;16:661-670.
7. Koller BH, Kim HS, Latour AM, Brigman K, Boucher RC, Jr., Scambler P, Wainwright B, Smithies O. Toward an animal model of cystic fibrosis: Targeted interruption of exon 10 of the cystic fibrosis transmembrane regulator gene in embryonic stem cells. *Proc Natl Acad Sci USA* 1991;88:10730-10734.
8. Rosenfeld MA, Yoshimura K, Trapnell BC, Yoneyama K, Rosenthal ER, Dalemans W, Fukayama M, Bargon J, Stier LE, Stratford-Perricaudet L, Perricaudet M, Guggino WB, Pavirani A, Lecocq JP, Crystal RG. *In vivo* transfer of the human cystic fibrosis

transmembrane conductance regulator gene to the airway epithelium. *Cell* 1992;68:143-155.

9. Miller JB, Boyer EH. A nontoxic detergent for aerosol use in dissolving viscid bronchopulmonary secretions. *J Pediat* 1952;40:767-771.
10. Chernick WS, Barbero GJ. Composition of tracheobronchial secretions in cystic fibrosis of the pancreas and bronchiectasis. *Pediatrics* 1959;24:739-745.
11. Matthews LW, Spector S, Lemm J, Potter J. Studies on Pulmonary Secretions: I. The over-all chemical composition of pulmonary secretions from patients with cystic fibrosis, bronchiectasis, and laryngectomy. *Am Rev Resp Dis* 1963;88:199-204.
12. Chernick WS, Barbero GJ, Eichel HJ. *In-vitro* evaluation of effect of enzymes on tracheobronchial secretions from patients with cystic fibrosis. *Pediatrics* 1961;27:589-596.
13. Shak S, Capon DJ, Hellmiss R, Marster SA, Baker CL. Recombinant human DNase I reduces the viscosity of cystic fibrosis sputum. *Proc Natl Acad Sci USA* 1990;87:9188-9192.
14. Kessler WR, Andersen DH. Heat prostration in fibrocystic disease of the pancreas and other conditions. *Pediatrics* 1951;8:648-656.
15. di Sant'Agnese PA, Darling RC, Perera GA, Shea E. Abnormal electrolyte composition of sweat in cystic fibrosis of the pancreas: Clinical significance and relationship to the disease. *Pediatrics* 1953;12:549-563.
16. Drumm ML, Pope HA, Cliff WH, Rommens JM, Marvin SA, Tsui LC, Collins FS, Frizzell RA, Wilson JM. Correction of the cystic fibrosis defect *in vitro* by retrovirus-mediated gene transfer. *Cell* 1990;62:1227-1233.
17. Kaiser D, Pivetta O, Rennert OM. Autosomal recessively inherited electrolyte excretory defect in the parotid of the "cribriform degeneration" mouse mutant--Possible analogy to cystic fibrosis. *Life Sci* 1974;15:803-810.
18. Martinez JR. Overview of animal models for cystic fibrosis. in Martinez JR, Barbero GJ (eds) *Animal Models for Cystic Fibrosis: The Reserpine-treated Rat*. San Francisco: San Francisco Press, 1985.
19. Grondin G, Leblond FA, Morisset J, Lebel D. Light and electron microscopy of the exocrine pancreas in the chronically reserpinized rat. *Pediatr Res* 1989;25:482-489.
20. Eppig JJ, Leiter EH. Exocrine pancreatic insufficiency syndrome in CBA/J mice: I. Ultrastructural study. *Am J Pathol* 1977;86:17-30.
21. Leiter EH, Dempsey EC, Eppig JJ. Exocrine pancreatic insufficiency syndrome in CBA/J mice: II. Biochemical studies. *Am J Pathol* 1977;86:31-43.
22. McPherson MA, Dormer RL. Molecular basis of cystic fibrosis. *Molec Asp Med* 1991;12:1-81.
23. Forstner J, Roomi N, Fahim R, Gall G, Perdue M, Forstner G. Acute and chronic models for hypersecretion of intestinal mucin. *Ciba Found Symp* 1984;97:61-71.
24. Martinez JR, Martinez AM. The reserpine-treated rat as an experimental animal model for cystic fibrosis: Abnormal Cl transport in pancreatic acinar cells. *Pediatr Res* 1988;24:427-432.
25. Veeze HJ, Sinaasappel M, Bijman J, de Jonge HR. Ussing-chamber studies of large intestine of the chronically reserpinized rat (CRR). *Pediatr Pulmon Sup 4* 1989:119.
26. Snouwaert JN, Brigman KK, Latour AM, Malouf NN, Boucher RC, Smithies O, Koller BH. An animal model for cystic fibrosis made by gene targeting. *Science* 1992;257:1083-1088.
27. Collins FS, Wilson JM. A welcome animal model. *Nature* 1992;358:708-709.

28. Clarke LL, Grubb BR, Gabriel SE, Smithes O, Koller BH, Boucher RC. Defective epithelial transport in a gene-targeted mouse model of cystic fibrosis. *Science* 1992;257:1125-1128.

Update: Duchenne Muscular Dystrophy and Myoblast Transfer

Eric Dunayer

"Scientific Problems with Animal Models of Duchenne Muscular Dystrophy" (Volume 3, *Perspectives on Medical Research*) discussed myoblast-transfer research (both *in vitro* and *in vivo*) aimed at uncovering a treatment for Duchenne muscular dystrophy (DMD).[1] In such research, immature muscle cells (myoblasts) are injected into diseased muscle with the hope that they will fuse to the muscle's cells and produce the muscle protein dystrophin, which is lacking or dysfunctional in DMD patients. This dystrophin production may then prevent muscle necrosis, seen in DMD.

Myoblast transfer was first achieved *in vitro*.[2] Following this success, researchers tested the technique in nonhuman-animals. Although myoblast transfer supposedly prevented muscle necrosis in *dy/dy*^{2j} mice,[3] who ordinarily develop a fatal muscular dystrophy, pathologist Terence A. Partridge has questioned this finding. In *dy/dy*^{2j} mice, muscle necrosis has a neurologic, not muscular, cause. How, then, could this necrosis be prevented by myoblast transfer, which compensates for a *muscle* defect?[4] Researchers also tried the technique in *mdx* mice, a strain that suffers spontaneous muscle necrosis due to an absence of dystrophin. In these mice, myoblast transfer apparently restored muscle function.[2,4] Again, however, experimental validity is highly doubtful. Unlike DMD patients, *mdx* mice show complete, spontaneous muscle regeneration following initial muscle necrosis, with little or no permanent muscle weakness.[2,4] Because irradiation prevents this normal recovery, researchers irradiated the mice before performing myoblast transfer.[2,4] Both the disease's normal course in the mice and the irradiation, therefore, constituted undermining variables--elements entirely absent in DMD. Finally, researchers tried myoblast transfer in CXMD dogs, a strain of golden retrievers whose muscles lack dystrophin.[5] In one experiment, the dogs showed signs of rejecting the transferred myoblasts, even though the dogs were administered immunosuppressants.[5] In another experiment, the myoblasts did fuse with the abnormal muscle (likely, administering higher doses of immunosuppressants to the dogs prevented myoblast rejection); the myoblasts, however, failed to produce dystrophin.[5]

Disregarding the nonhuman-animal data's inconsistency and apparent invalidity, researchers proceeded with human clinical trials. Initially they reported encouraging outcomes.[4]

Since the publication of "Scientific Problems with Animal Models of Duchenne Muscular Dystrophy," however, the clinical results of myoblast transfer have proved contradictory and suspect. Peter Law and his colleagues have reported promising results in DMD patients receiving myoblast transfer,[6,7] but other research groups have failed to duplicate these results.[6,7] Further, some researchers have questioned Law's methods of data collection and reporting (for example, his acknowledged exclusion of some test results that indicated lack of improvement in DMD patients); an FDA investigation has resulted.[6,7]

Following a 1992 conference on myoblast transfer, 25 researchers in the field of muscle development and disease wrote a letter to *Science* urging a temporary halt to all studies involving myoblast transfer as a treatment for children with DMD. Such studies, the researchers stated, "indicate only limited survival of the implanted myoblasts and no significant improvement in the clinical status of these children." The anesthesia and immunosuppressants used in the procedure, the researchers noted, place DMD patients at unacceptable risk. They advocated that clinical trials involving myoblast transfer cease until further animal studies have supplied more data.[7]

Additional animal research, however, is unlikely to clarify the prospects of treating DMD with myoblast transfer. To date, myoblast-transfer studies in nonhuman animals have provided conflicting results compromised by species differences in immunology, muscular physiology, and pathology.

References

1. Dunayer E. Scientific problems with animal models of Duchenne muscular dystrophy. *Perspec Med Res* 1991;3:1-21.
2. Partridge T. Use of normal myogenic cells to repair, replace, and rescue *mdx* mouse muscle from necrosis, in Angelini C, Danieli GA, Fontanari D (eds): *Muscular Dystrophy Research: From Molecular Diagnosis toward Therapy*. New York, Excerpta Medica, 1991.
3. Law PK, Goodwin TG, Li HJ, Ajamoughli G, Chen M. Myoblast transfer improves muscle genetics/structure/function and normalizes the behavior and life span of dystrophic mice, in Griggs R, Karpati G (eds). *Myoblast Transfer Therapy*. New York, Plenum Press, 1990.
4. Partridge TA. Myoblast transfer. A possible therapy for inherited myopathies? *Muscle & Nerve* 1991;14:197-212.
5. Discussion of Drs. Kornegay's, Bartlett's, and Cooper's papers, in Griggs R, Karpati G (eds). *Myoblast Transfer Therapy*. New York, Plenum Press, 1990.
6. Thompson L. Cell-transplant results under fire. *Science* 1992;257:472-474.
7. Thompson L. Researchers call for time out on cell-transplant research. *Science* 1992;257:738.

A New Method of Skin Research

Paul Contard

Traditionally, skin research has relied on three methods: animal models, tissue cultures, and mono-layer cell cultures (cells grown in a single layer on the bottom of a culture dish). All three research methods have serious drawbacks. Animal models are expensive, unreliable, and difficult to manipulate experimentally. Tissue cultures are often less inexpensive and more amenable to experimental manipulation than animal models, but microscopically they do not resemble normal tissue and often they do not synthesize the same substances as the normal tissues from which they were derived.

A newly developed cell-culture system in which skin cells are grown on a pre-treated nylon mesh[1] offers exciting possibilities. The technique uses human fibroblasts (cells that form connective tissue) derived from the dermis (lower skin layer). The fibroblasts are seeded into the mesh and allowed to grow in an incubator over several weeks. Cells from the epidermis (upper skin layer) are then seeded onto the cultured dermal cells and incubated for several more weeks. In cooperation with Advanced Tissue Sciences (Lajolla, CA), our laboratory has, over the past two years, studied this system's microscopic and biochemical aspects. Our findings have been highly encouraging.

In its microscopic features (as seen under both light and electron microscopes), this cell-culture system closely resembles normal human skin.[2,3] The system's cells, biochemical and histochemical (chemical composition determined by microscopy) analyses have shown, synthesize the same biological substances as normal human skin, in almost identical quantities -- including various types of collagen, laminin, and fibronectin.[4]

Most promising of all is the system's ability to grow an intact basement membrane completely in culture.[5] The basement membrane's major functions appear to include attaching the overlying epidermis to the underlying dermis and assisting the interaction between these two cell populations. The basement membrane is critical to the normal embryologic development of skin; its dysfunction contributes to several skin diseases characterized by blistering -- among them, epidermolysis bullosa and bullous pemphigoid. In addition, the basement membrane plays a crucial role in many other body tissues, including tissues of the lungs, kidneys, gastrointestinal tract, and circulatory system; some diseases of these tissues are associated with basement membrane abnormalities.

This new cell culture technology promises to revolutionize biomedical research. Already, it is being marketed for *in vitro* toxicology testing, and it may prove highly valuable for studying the course and treatment of a variety of skin diseases. Other tissues, such pancreatic, liver, and bone tissue,[6] also have been grown in laboratories using this new technology, which may soon render many areas of animal research totally obsolete.

References

1. Naughton G, Naughton BA. A physiologic skin model for *in vitro* toxicity studies, in Goldberg A (ed). *In Vitro Toxicology: New Directions*. New York, Mary A. Liebert, 1989.
2. Contard P, Jacobs L, Perlish JS, Fleischmajer R. Collagen fibrillogenesis in a three dimensional cell culture system. *Cell Tissue Res*, in press.
3. Fleischmajer R, Contard P, Schwartz E, MacDonald ED, Jacobs L, Sakai L. Elastin-associated microfibrils (10nm) in a three dimensional fibroblast culture. *J Invest Dermatol* 1991;97:638.
4. Fleischmajer R, MacDonald ED, Contard P, Perlish JS. Immunochemistry of a keratinocyte-fibroblast co-culture model for reconstructing human skin. *J Histochem Cytochem*, in press.
5. Contard P, Bartel RL, Jacobs JS, et al. Culturing keratinocytes and fibroblasts in a 3-dimensional mesh results in epidermal differentiation and formation of a basal lamina-anchoring zone. *J Invest Dermatol* 1993;100:35.
6. Rhonda Bartel, Director, epithelial cell culture development, Advanced Tissue Sciences, La Jolla, California, personal communication, 1991.

A Critique of Neurology Experiments at Northwestern University

Murry J. Cohen, Deborah N. Black, Roger S. Fouts, Frank W. Dobbs

In an attempt to gain information relevant to the neurological basis of human speech, Dr. Charles R. Larson, associate professor of Speech and Language Pathology in the Department of Communication Sciences and Disorders at Northwestern University, has, since 1978, served as principal investigator in invasive experiments that study "neural mechanisms of laryngeal control" in the pig-tailed macaque monkey (*Macaca nemestrina*). From April 1983 through March 1986, Larson's research was funded by a National Institutes of Health grant (cost unknown).[1] Larson requested a five year grant to continue this line of research, but it was funded for only three years, from April 1986 through March 1989, at a direct cost of $259,334 (indirect costs unknown).[1] This critique will focus on Larson's 1986-1991 grant request.

Summary of Larson's 1986-1991 Grant Proposal

Stated Aims

To study vocalization, Larson proposed investigating how, in monkeys, neuronal activity within the midbrain periaqueductal gray (PAG) and brainstem relates to laryngeal and respiratory muscles (intercostal and abdominal muscles, and the diaphragm).[1] In one group of monkeys, Larson would record PAG activity while monkeys vocalized, to determine whether stimulation of neurons within the nucleus ambiguus (NA, the site of laryngeal motoneurons) results in PAG activity. In a second group, he would stimulate NA neurons and record activity within the respiratory muscles. In a third group, he would trace nerve fibers to and from the PAG via neurochemical markers.[1]

Larson justified his project on these grounds: "It is important to study the neural control of vocalization in order to understand the human speech production process itself and to learn how neurologic disorders such as Huntington's Disease, Parkinsonism, and spastic dysphonia affect vocalization. . . . The present study will analyze the activity of different PAG neurons with respect to their projections to the nucleus ambiguus and muscles of the respiratory and laryngeal systems."[1]

Experimental Method and Procedure

For the period 1986-1991, Larson proposed using eight juvenile male pig-tailed macaque monkeys each year.[1] Six would be trained to vocalize for recording experiments; the two others would be used in neuroanatomical tracing studies. Those monkeys trained to vocalize would be food-deprived five days of each week and maintained at 90% of their normal weight. All monkeys would be caged alone.

During the experimental procedure itself, the monkeys would be placed, one at a time, in a primate restraining chair located in a sound-proof room. Apple juice would reinforce vocalization. A tube to deliver the juice reward, a microphone, and two lights that would serve as cues to vocalize would be located in front of each monkey.

During a 2-3 month training period, the monkeys would be taught to enter the restraining chair where, for 1-2 hours each day, they would be conditioned to vocalize. If a monkey emitted a sufficiently loud and long vocalization, he would receive juice (via computer-regulated delivery).

Following training, each monkey would undergo three surgical procedures, with a two-week recovery period between each procedure and the next.

In the first surgical procedure, a patch of skin two centimeters in diameter would be removed from the back of the monkey's head; a plastic plug would then be fastened to the exposed skull, with screws and dental cement. If a monkey were being used to study the laryngeal muscles, an incision would be made down the center of his throat, sufficient tissue would be cut away to expose his larynx, and electrodes would be inserted into his laryngeal muscles. If, instead, a monkey were being used to study the respiratory muscles, his pectoralis major (a large chest muscle) would be severed from his sternum and, through a needle, electrodes would be inserted into his intercostal muscles (between the ribs) and diaphragm. Electrodes would similarly be placed into abdominal muscles through an abdominal incision.

In the second surgical procedure, each monkey would have his upper four neck vertebrae fused to his skull with screws and dental cement, to prevent head movement from interfering with the recording of muscle activity. Larson refers to this procedure as "standard."[1]

In the third surgical procedure, each monkey would have his "scalp removed and the underlying skull area scraped bare."[1] Screw holes would then be drilled in his skull, to which the chamber holding recording and stimulating electrodes would be fastened with screws and dental cement. Nuts would be fixed to the skull. During recording sessions, these nuts would be screwed into metal braces of the restraining chair, to hold the monkey's head rigid.

One week after the last surgical procedure, the experimental period would begin, anticipated to last 1-2 months for each monkey. Bound in the restraining chair, his head completely immobilized, a monkey would be required to vocalize for juice. Meanwhile, electrodes would record neuronal and muscular activity. After PAG neurons had been exhaustively explored for a given monkey, he would be anesthetized, then killed by electrical current passed through his brain. The body would then be perfused with formalin and the brain removed.

Critique of Larson's Experiments

Fundamental differences between monkey vocalization and human speech, as well as numerous confounding variables, render Larson's work inherently unsound and inapplicable to humans.

Differences between Monkey Vocalization and Human Speech

In many respects, monkey vocalization and human speech are *not* homologous. Whereas human vocalizations are generally produced voluntarily and controlled with great ease, monkey vocalizations seem largely dependent on the arousal of strong feeling in the monkey. Experiments on rhesus monkeys (*Macaca mulatta*) have indicated that their vocalizations usually signal intense feelings--such as alarm, hunger, or loneliness--relating to some basic need.[2] In contrast, humans routinely speak without, simultaneously, experiencing strong emotion. Larson himself acknowledges, "It has been suggested that human speech, being propositional in nature, is fundamentally different from most types of animal vocalizations."[3]

Researchers' difficulty in conditioning monkey species to vocalize on cue provides support for the view that monkey vocalization ordinarily has an affective basis. Although, in a study coauthored by Larson, researchers claimed that rhesus monkeys had learned to vocalize on cue,[4] Shun-Ichi Yamaguchi and Ronald Myers failed to elicit such conditioned vocalization. They concluded that rhesus monkeys may lack voluntary control of their vocalizations.[5] In the wild, rhesus monkeys produce at least 20 different calls, yet researchers have claimed success in conditioning rhesus monkeys to vocalize very few such sounds.

Larson's own work suggests that, in monkeys, the PAG links limbic-system areas and motor nuclei controlling laryngeal and respiratory muscles;[6] since the limbic system mediates emotion, this suggested link provides further evidence that monkey vocalization may be highly emotion-dependent. The PAG's role in vocalization, therefore, may be much more important in monkeys than in humans, in whom PAG function remains poorly defined. Larson admits, "If . . . it is only important for coordination of affective vocalizations, then the PAG may not be that crucial for normal [human] speech."[3]

Larson has also acknowledged that monkey vocalization and human speech may be "controlled by different neural mechanisms."[3] Anthropologist Gordon

Hewes has noted that "primate cries and calls are handled by parts of the cortex, bilaterally, some distance away from the lateralized [human] speech areas," which are "localized in an entirely different portion of the cortex."[7] Further, as Larson himself has noted, the human cortex extends neural projections to the nucleus ambiguus, whereas the monkey cortex does not.[3]

Confounding Variables

Metabolic, immunological, and other physiological changes induced by the stress of experimental procedures alter experimental measurements and confound results.[8] In monkeys, psychological stress has been shown to alter plasma cortisol levels, associated with neurotransmitter levels.[9] In Larson's experiments, the stress inflicted on the monkeys is intense. These profoundly social animals are isolated, subjected to multiple highly invasive surgical procedures, deprived of food, and forced to endure severe and prolonged immobilization. Surely, the monkeys experience substantial pain and fear.

The mere handling of monkeys can result in measurable physiological changes.[10] Pulse rates of rhesus monkeys change when humans enter the room.[11] Many monkeys find isolation so stressful that they develop self-mutilating behavior.[12] Immobilization stress, too, causes profound biological changes; in monkeys, immobilization "has repeatedly been shown to have major endocrinological and physiological repercussions," including effects on the autoimmune system.[13] In non-human animals, the PAG is known to interact with brain structures that are profoundedly influenced by stress levels, including pain sensitivity and blood pressure.[14] Therefore, it is likely that laboratory stress will confound the research results.

Lack of Clinical Relevance

Larson claims that his research will help us gain insight into the process whereby human neurological disorders such as Huntington's disease (HD), Parkinson's disease (PD), and spastic dysphonia (SD) affect vocalization. A number of neurologists, neurobiologists, and neuropsychologists who have reviewed Larson's work have disputed this claim, which seems untenable.[15] HD, PD, and SD--chronic, degenerative illnesses--have anatomical, chemical, and physiological characteristics that have never been faithfully reproduced in animals.[16] Larson's research appears to have little relevance to these neurologic diseases. For example, both HD and PD result from loss of neurons, with consequent biochemical deficiency, in brain areas different from those that Larson is studying.[16]

Alternatives to Animal Experimentation

Major advances in understanding HD, PD, and SD have derived from clinical research and from human gene-mapping (tracing correlations between the existence of abnormal genes and the occurrence of disease).[16,17] Such research has led to improved prevention through genetic counseling.

Increasingly, clinical research on neurological diseases involves sophisticated computer technologies. For example, Positron Emission Tomography (PET) scans show which portions of the brain come into play during a particular activity (such as vocalization); these scans now yield three-dimensional images offering a resolution of about four millimeters in the brainstem. PET scanning and other computerized imaging techniques provide a non-invasive means of obtaining highly precise information regarding the functional relationships between the cortex and brainstem in human vocalization. The Institute of Medicine's Committee on a National Neural Circuitry Database recommends the use of such computerized techniques,[18] which have obvious and important advantages over animal experimentation: these techniques cause no suffering, are both valid and precise, and are directly relevant to human health.

Summary and Conclusion

The results of experiments that investigate monkey vocalizations are unlikely to apply to human speech. Whereas monkey vocalization appears highly dependent on the arousal of strong feeling, humans routinely speak without strong emotion. Monkey vocalization and human speech also differ significantly in their underlying neural circuitry.

The monkeys used in Larson's experiments are subjected to such extreme stress that any obtained data are further invalidated by such confounding variables as undetermined changes in metabolism, immunology, and other physiological parameters. Along with interspecies differences, such variables preclude the possibility of clarifying the PAG's role in human speech.

It is highly improbable that Larson's type of animal experimentation can provide insight into how HD, PD, SD, and other human neurological disorders affect speech. The greatest advances in understanding, treating, and preventing these diseases have derived from clinical research and clinical intervention, including advanced imaging technologies, population studies, human gene-mapping, and genetic counseling.

References

1. Neural Mechanisms of Laryngeal Control. Federal grant application PHS 2 RO1 NS19290-04, April 1, 1986-March 31, 1991, Charles R. Larson, principal investigator.

2. Myers RE. Comparative neurology of vocalization and speech: Proof of a dichotomy, in Harnad SR, Steklis HD, Lancaster J (eds). *Origins and Evolution of Language and Speech.* New York Academy of Sciences 1976;280:745-757.
3. Larson CR. The midbrain periaqueductal gray: A brainstem structure involved in vocalization. *J Speech Hearing Res* 1985;28:241-249.
4. Sutton D, Larson C, Taylor EM, Lindeman RC. Vocalization in rhesus monkeys: Conditionability. *Brain Res* 1973;52:225-231.
5. Yamaguchi S-I, Myers RE. Failure of discriminative vocal conditioning in *Rhesus* monkey. *Brain Res* 1972;37:109-114.
6. Larson CR, Kistler MK. The relationship of periaqueductal gray neurons to vocalization and laryngeal EMG in the behaving monkey. *Exp Br Res* 1986;63:596-606.
7. Hewes G. The current status of the gestural theory of language origin, in Harnad SR, Steklis HD, Lancaster J (eds). *Origins and Evolution of Language and Speech.* New York Academy of Sciences 1976;280:482-504.
8. Barnard N, Hou S. Inherent stress--the tough life in lab routine. *Lab Animal* 1988;17: 21-27.
9. Hill CW, Greer WE, Felsenfeld O. Psychological stress, early response to foreign protein, and blood cortisol in vervets. *Psychosom Med* 1967;29:279-283.
10. Fox MW. *Laboratory Animal Husbandry Ethology Welfare and Experimental Variables.* Albany, SUNY Pr, 1986.
11. Malinow MR, Hill JD, Ochsner AJ. Heart rate in caged rhesus monkeys (*Macaca mulatta*). *Lab An Sci* 1974;24:537-540.
12. Crawley JN, Sutton ME, Pickar D. Animal models of self-destructive behavior and suicide. *Psychol Clin NA* 1985;8:299-310.
13. Katsiia GV, Todua TN, Gorlushkin VM, et al. Effect of immobilization stress on gonadotropic function of the hypophysis in male hamadryas baboons (*Papio hamadrysas*). *Biull Eskp Biol Med* 1989;107:231-234.
14. Bandler R, Carrive P, Zhang SP. Integration of somatic and autonomic reactions within the midbrain pariaquaductal grey: Visceral, somatotopic, and functional organization. *Prog Br Res* 1991;87:269-305.
15. *Charles R. Larson, Northwestern University, Grant #2 R01 NS19290-04*, Section 2: Independent Evaluations of the Grant. Concerned Citizens for Ethical Research, Evanston, 1991.
16. Kaufman SR, Czarnecki T, Haralabatos I, Richardson M. Animal models of degenerative neurological diseases. *Perspec Med Res* 1991;3:9-48.
17. Henreen JC, Zweig RM, DeLong MR, Whitehouse PJ, Price DL. Primary dystonias: A review of the pathology and suggestions for new directions of study. *Adv Neurol* 1988;50:123-132.
18. Pechura CM, Martin JB (eds). *Mapping The Brain And Its Functions.* National Academy Press, Washington, D.C., 1991.

Critique of an Animal Model for Testing the Anti-Anxiety Potential of the Experimental Drug NO-328

Murry J. Cohen

Introduction

Dr. James E. Barrett is attempting to study the anxiolytic (anti-anxiety or tranquilizing) properties of an experimental drug called NO-328 by observing its effects in squirrel monkeys. His research is being conducted at The Uniformed Services University of the Health Sciences, in cooperation with the Henry M. Jackson Foundation for the Advancement of Military Medicine. The project is entitled *Experimental Assessment of NO-328: A GABA-Uptake Inhibitor with Potential Anxiolytic Activity.*[1] Extramural support was provided by NOVO Industri A/S, to whom "any material stemming from the conduct of these experiments will first be submitted."[1]

Purpose of the Proposed Experiment

The major anxiolytic drugs currently available are the benzodiazepines, such as diazepam or chlordiazepoxide. These drugs work by chemically altering a specific receptor present on neuronal cell membranes, a reaction that involves the neurotransmitter gama-aminobutyric acid (GABA). Benzodiazepines act immediately and show great efficacy in reducing anxiety. However, they may produce certain undesirable effects, such as sedation, impaired cognition, potentiation (magnification of the effects) of other central nervous system depressants, and development of tolerance, dependence, and addiction.[2]

A newer type of anxiolytic is bupropion, a serotonergic drug that works by increasing the level of the neurotransmitter serotonin in the nervous system. Less is known about this drug's effectiveness than that of the benzodiazepines. Bupropion can require several weeks before taking effect, and the side-effects in some patients can be unpleasant. Furthermore, its efficacy is reduced in many patients previously treated with benzodiazepines. It does not, however, seem to result in tolerance and dependence.

In an attempt to find a useful anxiolytic drug without the disadvantages of the benzodiazepines and serotonergics, Barrett is studying drugs with different mechanisms of action. One such drug is NO-328 (R-(-)-1-(4,4-(3-methyl-2-thienyl)-3-piperidine carboxylic acid hydrochloride), whose mechanism of action seems different from that of the two classes of currently available anxiolytics. According to Barrett, this drug is "a potent and selective inhibitor of the uptake of ^{3}H-GABA [and] may represent a new type of anxiolytic, with its primary mechanism of action through the GABA system" rather than the benzodiazepine receptor system.[1] This means that the drug directly inhibits the enzymes that normally break down GABA, causing higher GABA concentrations in the nervous system, *without* necessarily interacting with the benzodiazepine receptor system. If GABA functions *directly* as an anxiolytic ligand, without requiring biochemical interaction with other benzodiazepine receptor chemicals, then NO-328 and related drugs might function as anxiolytics through a novel, safer, and more effective mechanism of action, and would represent a contribution to our drug arsenal.

Barrett reports that his experiment "is designed to examine the specific potential anxiolytic activity of NO-328 in a well-characterized and widely-accepted primate animal model for the detection of anxiolytic drugs. This model, which employs the maintenance of a selected response by periodic presentation of food, [followed by] suppression of that behavior by punishment, has been used extensively in behavioral pharmacology for studying anxiolytic drugs and correlates well with clinical efficacy."[1] Such reliance on animal experiments to explore the "behavioral pharmacology" of psychotropic drugs for potential application to human beings is indeed common.[3] Barrett himself has devoted much of career to such research, specifically investigation of the squirrel monkey's behavioral responses to pharmacologic interventions and has added to a large amount of data on this subject.[4]

Summary of the Proposed Experiment

Barrett's experimental paradigm consists of a commonly used laboratory procedure to test potentially anxiolytic drugs. In his experiment, six squirrel monkeys who have become adapted to a primate chair are to be taught to press a lever for food under both nonpunishment and punishment circumstances. Punishment, delivered by administering an electric shock to the monkeys' tails, has predictably been found to "suppress responding to [lever pressing] levels . . . below those normally occurring."[1] According to Barrett, "It is the performance under this condition . . . that provides the most meaningful information on whether a drug is or will be a clinically effective anxiolytic compound. All such drugs will increase this punished responding. . ."[1]

After the experimental sessions, the monkeys "are returned to their home living cages in a large colony room with visual and auditory access to other monkeys."[1] The anxiolytic and sedative effects of NO-328 are determined by analyzing the drug's effects on both punished and unpunished behavior. The anxiolytic effect is ascertained by seeing if the drug results in an increase in punished behavior, and the sedative effect is gauged by looking for a decrease in unpunished behavior.

The experimental drug is administered through a tube which, over the course of 1-2 minutes, is inserted into the monkeys' stomachs. Some of the monkeys will be given only placebos; in their case, the stress, anxiety, and apprehension brought on by the experimental procedure will definitely be unalleviated: "The compound under investigation may have stress alleviating actions, but monkeys will not always be administered this compound." Barrett assigns the "level of pain or distress to be imposed" a value of "three" on a scale of one to five.

Critique of the Proposed Experiment

Considering the difficulties encountered with the effective but problematic benzodiazepines and the less-than-optimally-effective serotonergic anxiolytics, the attempt to identify an improved anxiolytic drug is a worthwhile endeavor. The *subject* of Barrett's experiments is not trivial. His chosen methodology, however, warrants serious criticism into two categories: criticism of the animal model approach *per se* and criticism of other aspects of the experiment.

Criticism of the Animal Model Approach

Animal models have long been used to study human psychiatric illnesses,[5] despite numerous objections to this approach.[6-13] Promoters of animal experimentation have convinced much of the public that psychopharmacologic breakthroughs have derived directly from these experiments.[14] However, Reines' comprehensive historical review revealed that "The discoverers of modern psychopharmacology were clinical investigators who noted mood-altering side-effects of drugs used in clinical practice."[11]

Just as basic science investigators and animal experimenters have inappropriately claimed credit for many other medical breakthroughs,[15] they have claimed credit for the development of psychotropic drugs. A publication of the Foundation for Biomedical Research states that "medications to treat mental illness . . . required animal research in their development."[16] A former president of the American Psychiatric Association has written that "animal research has provided medicines for use against schizophrenia, depression, panic disorder, obsessive-compulsive disorder, and manic-depressive illness."[17] Such statements, however, "rewrite medical history."[12]

Let us examine the actual circumstances that led to the discovery of different classes of psychotropic drugs. Psychiatrist and neuroscientist Ross Baldessarini notes with respect to the phenothiazines: "Like most of the useful psychotropic agents, the effects of chlorpromazine were discovered by serendipitous clinical observation."[18] This fact is completely ignored by J.K. Krasney, who states that the development of chlorpromazine and its tranquilizing derivatives resulted from studies with rats, rabbits, and monkeys.[19]

Serendipity in Discovery of Benzodiazepines details Dr. Leo Sternbach's *in vitro* discovery of the first benzodiazepine anxiolytic, chlordiazepoxide, which was inspired by the chemical structure of chlorpromazine.[20] The tricyclic antidepressants were developed through clinical trials, after chlorpromazine's chemical structure inspired their synthesis.[11] The monoamine oxidase inhibiting antidepressants were discovered in a clinical context, when they were noted to result in euphoria during use in tuberculosis treatment.[21]

Writing in the *Comprehensive Textbook of Psychiatry*, psychiatrist John Davis sums up the case of psychotropic drugs: "Many of the psychotropic drugs were discovered by chance when they were administered for one indication and observed to be helpful for an entirely different condition. The history of the development of both the antidepressants and the antipsychotic drugs points up the fact that major medical discoveries can evolve as a consequence of clinical investigation, rather than deductions from basic animal research."[13]

In the case of newer psychotropic medications as well, animal models have played neither a generative nor a crucial developmental role. In the case of bupropion, "a clinical hypothesis prompted the animal modelers' work."[11] With fluoxetine, *in vitro* studies demonstrated its selective inhibition of serotonin uptake.[22] While the standard animal tests failed to predict anti-depressant effects, human clinical trials demonstrated its value for depression therapy.[23]

The development of lithium as a psychotropic illustrates such clinical discovery. Although some proponents of animal experimentation have promoted the view that John Cade's discovery of lithium's anti-manic effects was preceded by crucial animal experimentation,[17,24] Cade's work with animals actually *followed* this discovery. Cade first learned of lithium's anti-manic effects in 19th century clinical reports of patients whose "gouty mania" was relieved by lithium salts.[24-26] The subsequent animal experiments merely dramatized the clinical findings and "sold" them to skeptical scientists.[11,15,27]

Data from animal model work has, in fact, been notoriously misleading in our efforts to understand psychoactive drugs. Animal experiments failed to identify the addictive potential of pentazocine (the use of which was eventually curtailed), the amnesic effect of triazolam (which underwent an altered dosage recommendation after years of clinical use), the abuse/addictive potential of methaqualone (eventually withdrawn), the overdose dangers of glutethemid (eventually withdrawn), or the lethality of nomifensine (eventually withdrawn).

In the case of anxiolytics, the abuse potential of the benzodiazepines was not revealed in animal studies. It took years of clinical use to reveal the substantial addictive properties of this class of drugs, which were due to their tendency to induce tolerance and dependence in chronic users. For example, Alprazolam is particulary addictive, in part because its duration of action is short. Animal studies, however, did not predict alprazolam's highly addictive potential.

Animal models have contributed little or nothing to the development of psychotropic medications. There is no reason to think that Barrett's use of the animal model in an effort to discover a new type of anxiolytic will prove an exception.

Considering all the drawbacks and inadequacies of the animal model, why does such an experimental method continue to be proposed and funded? Barrett himself provides a partial explanation with his comment that this method has been "extensively used . . . for studying anxiolytic drugs."[1] It is common for proponents of animal models to justify their use on the grounds that they have been used in the past. Given today's sophistication in computer manipulation and mathematical modelling,[28] and the degree of success of *in vitro* and clinical research methods in developing psychotropic drugs, Barrett's nonhuman animal behavioral paradigm seems both archaic and inexcusable.

Scientific Problems with the Animal Model

The animal model approach to drug investigation is inherently invalid; experiments on nonhuman animals do not yield data that can be extrapolated to humans.[29-31] Animal models differ from human conditions in several critical respects, including their means of induction, their natural histories, and, most fundamentally, in the species in which the condition occurs. Consequently, there are differences between the animals' condition and any "analogous" human condition in anatomy, physiology, and pathology that make animal data difficulty, if not impossible, to interpret in terms of *human* disease.

Problems with animal models are perhaps most obvious in psychological research. Difficulties communicating with nonhuman animals undermine all efforts to understand animal psychology. Laboratory studies are particularly inappropriate, because it is impossible to interpret the psychological status of animals whose behavior is altered by the unnatural laboratory environment and whose normal psychology is profoundly altered by experimental manipulations that have no meaningful correlation to the natural environment in which the animals evolved. Furthermore, Barrett's lever-pressing, tail-shocking tests illustrate these problems well. It is impossible to guage NO-328's precise effect on the monkeys. If the monkeys given the drug show increased lever-pressing, is this because the drug has acted as a pain-killer? An appetite stimulant? A tranquilizer? Has the drug merely induced hyperactivity? These questions can't be answered.

Further, animals experience hormonal, immunological, and neurological changes caused by the stress of being in a laboratory; these changes alter measurements and confound results[32]--precluding the discovery of useful findings. In monkeys and other primates, immobilization stress alone "has repeatedly been shown to have major endocrinological and physiological repercussions for the organism, including autoimmune disorders."[33] Barrett's experiment creates severe distress by isolating inherently social animals, restraining them in a chair, shocking them, and traumatizing them with the insertion of a nasogastric tube. The pain and distress level induced by these conditions, which Barrett himself rates as "3" on a scale of one to five,[1] would produce sufficient changes in enzymatic, antibody, and neurotransmitter functions to render any obtained data invalid.

Conclusion

Barrett's lever-pressing animal "model" cannot assess the clinical efficacy of anxiolytic drugs. His research illustrates difficulties with animal models in general and animal use in psychology in particular. Progress in the pharmacological management of anxiety will occur where advances in psychology have always occurred -- in the clinical setting, where careful observation of drug effects on human mood and mentation have been responsible for psychiatric drug discoveries.

References

1. Barrett JE (principal investigator). Experimental Assessment of No-328: A GABA-Uptake Inhibitor With Potential Anxiolytic Activity. Federal grant application G18866-01.
2. Salzman C. The APA Task Force report on benzodiazepine dependence, toxicity and abuse (editorial). *Am J Psychiat* 1991;148:151-152.
3. Sepinwall J, Cook L. Behavioral pharmacology of antianxiety drugs, in Iversen LL, Iversen SD, Snyder SH (eds). *Handbook of Psychopharmacology, Vol. 13.* Plenum Press, New York, 1978, pp 345-393.
4. Barrett JE. Behavioral pharmacology of the squirrel monkey, in Rosenblum LA and Coe CL (eds): *Handbook of Squirrel Monkey Research.* Plenum Press, New York, 1985, pp 315-348.
5. Keehn JD. *Animal Models for Psychiatry.* Routledge & Kegan Paul, London (Methuen, New York), 1986.
6. Sitaram N, Gershon S. From animal models to clinical testing -- promises and pitfalls. *Prog Neuro-Psychopharmacol & Biol Psychiat* 1983;7:227-228.
7. Cohen, MJ. The irrelevance of animal experimentation in modern psychiatry and psychology, in Natelson NB, Cohen MJ (eds): *Proceedings of The First International Medical Conference "Future Medical Research Without The Use of Animals: Facing The Challenge."* (Held in Tel Aviv, Israel, May 15-16, 1990.) Concern for Helping Animals in Israel, Alexandria, Virginia, 1991.
8. Cohen, MJ. Animal testing (letter). *Psychiatric News*, November 20, 1987.
9. Barnes D. The use of nonhuman animals in psychobiological and behavioral research, in Natelson NB, Cohen MJ (eds): *Proceedings of The First International Medical Conference "Future Medical Research Without The Use of Animals: Facing The Challenge."* (Held in Tel Aviv, Israel, May 15-16, 1990.) Concern for Helping Animals in Israel, Alexandria, Virginia, 1991.
10. Barnes D. Animal models (letter). *Nature* 1987;329:666.
11. Reines, BP. Psychopharmacologic discovery: The relative contributions of clinical and laboratory studies. *Perspec Med Res* 1990;2:13-26.
12. Reines BP. Animal rights and research (letter). *Am J Psychiat* 1988;145:539-540.

13. Davis JM. Antipsychotic drugs, in Kaplan HI, Sadock BJ (eds): *Comprehensive Textbook of Psychiatry*, Fourth Edition, Williams & Wilkins, Baltimore, 1985.
14. Campion FD. *The AMA and U.S. Health Policy since 1940.* Chicago Rev Pr, Chicago, 1984.
15. Reines B. The process of medical discovery, in Natelson NB, Cohen MJ (eds): *Proceedings of The First International Medical Conference "Future Medical Research Without The Use of Animals: Facing The Challenge."* (Held in Tel Aviv, Israel, May 15-16, 1990.) Concern for Helping Animals in Israel, Alexandria, Virginia, 1991.
16. *The Use of Animals in Biomedical Research and Testing.* Foundation for Biomedical Research, June 1988.
17. Pardes H. "Dear Colleague" letter sent to all American Psychiatric Association members, November 1989.
18. Baldessarini RJ. Antipsychotic agents. *The Psychiatric Times*, Jan 1988.
19. Krasney JK. Some thoughts on the value of life. *Buffalo Physician* 1984;18:6-13.
20. Anon. Serendipity in discovery of benzodiazepines. *The Psychiatric Times*, Sep 1986.
21. Lehman H, Kline NS. Clinical discoveries with antidepressant drugs, in Parnham MJ, Bruinvels J (eds): *Discoveries in Pharmacology: Volume 1, Psycho- and Neuro-pharmacology.* Elsevier, New York, 1983.
22. Lemberger L, Farid NA, Bergstrom RF, Wolen RL. Fluoxetine, pharmacology and physiologic disposition. *Inter J Obesity* 1987;11(Suppl 3):157-161.
23. Lemberger L, Terman S, Rowe H, Billings R. The effects of nisoxetine (Lilly compound 94939), a potential antidepressant, on biogenic amine uptake in man. *Br J Clin Pharmacol* 1976;3:215-220.
24. Cade J. Lithium salts for the treatment of psychotic excitement. *Med J Austr* 1949;36: 349-351.
25. Johnson FN. *The History of Lithium Therapy*. London, Macmillan, 1984.
26. Reines BP. The relationship between laboratory and clinical studies in psychopharmacologic discovery. *Perspec Med Res* 1990;2:13-26.
27. Reines BP. On the locus of medical discovery. *The Journal of Medicine and Philosophy* 1991;16:183-209.
28. Bross ID. Mathematical models vs. animal models. *Perspec An Res* 1989;1:83-108.
29. Reines BP. A critique of animal psychology research at the University of California at Berkeley. *Perspec An Res* 1989;1:25-55.
30. Bannister D. The myth of physiological psychology. *Bull Br Psychol Soc* 1968;21:229-231.
31. Shuttlesworth DS, Neill D, Ellen P. The place of physiological psychology in neuroscience. *Physiological Psychology* 1984;12:3.
32. Barnard N, Hou S. Inherent stress -- the tough life in lab routine. *Lab Animal* 1988;17:21-27.
33. Katsiia GV, Todua TN, Gorlushkin VM, et al. Effect of immobilization stress on gonadotropic function of the hypophysis in male hamadryas baboons (*Papio hamadrysas*). *Biull Eskp Biol Med* 1989;107:231-234.

A Critique of Brain Mapping Experiments Using Animals at the Uniformed Services University of the Health Sciences

Murry J. Cohen

Human brain mapping reveals which brain regions receive sensory information from specific parts of the body. In cases of injury or congenital malformation, brain mapping elucidates the process by which an area of the brain that previously received information from the now-incapacitated body part adapts by developing sensory input from a different body party. This type of brain mapping is known as somatosensory tracking; one of its goals is to study cortical plasticity, the brain's ability to change function.

When performed in a clinically relevant manner--non-invasively, minimizing stress, and only on the species intended to be helped by the experiment's results--brain mapping can be extremely useful. In contrast, invasive animal experiments, such as those conducted by Dr. Sharon Juliano at the Uniformed Services University of the Health Sciences, have not advanced our understanding of human neuroanatomy, neurophysiology, or neuropathology. In Juliano's experiments, cats, kittens, and squirrel monkeys are subjected to the amputation of a digit, surgical brain damage, and other forms of neurological destruction.[1]

Setting complex scientific considerations aside for the moment, the sick and debilitated condition of Juliano's animals suffices to preclude the generation of meaningful data.[2-5] Of the ten monkeys used in the experiments, three died within a day of experimental brain surgery.[2-4] Post-mortem examination revealed the appalling condition of these animals. One was infested with abdominal parasites, dehydrated, and emaciated ("no fat stores");[2] another showed parasitic infection in the colon and lungs;[3] the third had suffered from intestinal parasites and heart disease.[4] In addition, two of the monkeys had previously undergone abdominal surgery:[3-5] one was missing a spleen;[5] the other, his left adrenal gland and kidney.[4] Why were such debilitated animals subjected to surgery? Why was this the *second* surgery for two of the animals? Surely, such methods are neither humane nor scientifically sound.

Even if the animals had been healthy, the hormonal and immunological changes produced by the stress of being in a laboratory would have precluded the possibility of valid findings. In an interview published in *The Washington Post*, Juliano stated, "we are not hurting the animals";[6] however, in her grant application she assigned the "level of pain and distress to be imposed on the animals" a value of 3 on a scale of 1-5.[1] Pain and distress alter measurements and confound results because of stress-induced physiological changes.[7] The stress induced merely by the unnatural isolation of these social animals would produce changes in neurotransmitter functions that alter experimental results.

In addition to the problems of disease and stress, Juliano's species choices seem arbitrary and nonscientific. Data from two different species, squirrel monkeys and cats, are to be applied to yet a third species, humans. Will results from the two different species be combined? If the results conflict, which will be considered more valid? If the results agree, to what extent will they apply to humans? It is impossible to know.

Why were cats selected as experimental subjects? Juliano offers four reasons, without once discussing generalizability and applicability to humans.[8] First, cats have *previously* been used in similar brain-mapping research; second, cats have been used in other types of brain-mapping research, such as amblyopia experiments (see pages 39-51 for a critique of such experiments); third, certain brain areas of interest are more "exposed" in cats than in other nonhuman animals, facilitating study; fourth, "the metabolic modular organization of the cat somatosensory cortex has not yet been studied in detail."[8] These four considerations are not appropriate justification for using cats as models for human beings.

Juliano cites prior visual deprivation experiments in which animals, usually cats, were deprived of sight by being blinded, having their eyelids sutured shut, or being kept in darkness. Purportedly, these experiments were conducted to elucidate "lazy eye syndrome" (amblyopia) in humans. Although Juliano does not study sight deprivation, she cites these experiments demonstrating central nervous system plasticity as precursors to her own.[1] But many vision scientists[9-11]--including von Noorden,[12] world-renowned in the field of sight deprivation and an advocate of animal experimentation--have criticized such animal studies because of the neuroanatomic and neurophysiologic differences between cats and humans. (In "amblyopia" research on cats, one major problem is that amblyopia is a disease involving the fovea centralis of the human retina, and the retina of cats contains no such structure.) Juliano completely ignores such interspecies differences.

Why did Juliano choose squirrel monkeys? It is often assumed that all primates closely resemble one another with respect to the parts of the brain that receive signals from specific parts of the body and that monkeys are, therefore, valid models for humans. However, squirrel monkeys differ considerably from owl monkeys in the cortical representations of body surfaces.[13] On what scientific grounds, then, can anyone assume that squirrel monkeys do not differ even more substantially from humans?

Juliano's grant proposal contains no mention of any possible clinical relevance of her work to humans. Only in a paper published in 1990, four years after she received her original NIH grant, does she indicate that her research may possibly advance our understanding of Alzheimer's disease.[14] The connection between Juliano's research and Alzheimer's Disease is, to say the least, vague and unconvincing.

Juliano completely ignores new, important, and technologically sophisticated advances in studying brain structure and function in humans--the CT, PET, and MRI scans. These imaging techniques, which offer means of directly studying the brains of people with peripheral neurological damage, are safe and non-invasive, provide diagnostic information that can directly help patients who participate in research protocols, and circumvent the problem of interspecies differences that renders animal experimentation scientifically unsound. In a recent monograph published by the National Academy of Sciences entitled *Mapping The Brain And Its Functions*, the Committee on a National Neural Circuitry Database of the Institute of Medicine acknowledged that "graphic depictions have proved to be so useful that greater and greater attention is being paid to the concept of visualization computing in biomedical sciences."[15]

Juliano's method of neuroscience research represents the antithesis of scientific investigation that is modern, reliable, accurate, and cost-effective. The archaic use of animal models in brain mapping should cease. Juliano's $376,829 in federal funding, and the millions of additional tax dollars spent on similar research, should be redirected to human studies with a genuine capacity to advance knowledge of neurological function and disease and thereby assist in improving people's health.

References

1. Juliano SL (principal investigator). Structural Correlates of Cortical Information Processing. Federal grant application PHS NS-24014, Jul 1, 1989-Jun 30, 1992.
2. Pathology Report, LAM Necropsy No. P-1-88, USUHS Pathology No. 88-37, Jul 31, 1989.
3. Pathology Report, LAM Necropsy No. P-3-90, USUHS Pathology No. 90-473, Dec 3, 1990.
4. Pathology Report, LAM Necropsy No. P-4-90, USUHS Pathology No. 90-482, Dec 21, 1990.
5. USUHS document dated Oct 7, 1991, signed by HC Holloway (Deputy Dean, School of Medicine), and provided to In Defense of Animals.
6. Anon. Protesters stalk researcher. *The Washington Post*, June 23, 1991.
7. Barnard N, Hou S. Inherent stress--the tough life in lab routine. *Lab Animal* 1988;17:21-27.
8. Juliano SL, Whitsel BL, Tommerdahl M, Cheema SS. Determinants of patchy metabolic labeling in the somatosensory cortex of cats: A possible role for intrinsic inhibitory circuitry. *J Neurosci* 1989;9:1-12.
9. Buyukmihci NC. Response to Dr. Blakemore's assertion that work involving nonhuman animals has led to significantly greater understanding and treatment of amblyopia. *Perspec An Res* 1989;1:57-62.
10. Abraham SV. A tribute to Claud Worth. *Ann Ophthalmol* 1972;4:171-175.
11. Marg E. Prentice Memorial Lecture: Is the animal model for stimulus deprivation amblyopia in children valid or useful? *Am J Optomet Physiol Optics* 1982;59:451-464.

12. von Noorden GK. Application of basic research data to clinical amblyopia. *Ophthalmology* 85:496-504;1978.

13. Jenkins WM, Merzenich MM. Reorganization of neocortical representations after brain injury: A neurophysiological model of the bases of recovery from stroke. *Prog Br Res* 1987;71:249-266.

14. Juliano SL, Bear MF, Eslin D. Cholinergic manipulation alters stimulus-evoked metabolic activity in cat somatosensory cortex. *J Comp Neurology* 1990;297:106-120.

15. Pechura CM, Martin JB (eds). *Mapping The Brain And Its Functions*. Washington, DC, National Academy Press, 1991.

The Clinical Relevance of Dr. Colin Blakemore's Vision Research

Stephen R. Kaufman, Deanna Z. Macek, Marvin Kraushar

Terminology:

amblyopia -- loss of vision in an eye due to disuse of that eye; while amblyopia is reversible during early childhood, most amblyopia that persists beyond childhood becomes permanent

anisometropia -- difference in refractive states of the two eyes; in other words, difference between the eyes in the lens power needed to focus light on the retina

ocular dominance of cortical neurons -- greater response of cortical brain neurons to light coming from one eye compared to the other eye, determined by firing rates of individual neurons as recorded by microelectrodes

strabismus -- misalignment of the eyes; also known as "squint" and "crossed eyes"

Dr. Colin Blakemore's visual deprivation research has generated ongoing controversy in England. Animal protectionists have charged that Blakemore's research is cruel to animals and irrelevant to humans.[1-3] A leading advocate of animal research,[4] Blakemore has countered that his research is important to the management of amblyopia, a leading cause of uniocular visual deficit.[5] As ophthalmologists, we will attempt to determine whether Blakemore's claim is supported by fact.

In order to assess Blakemore's claim that his research is clinically relevant, we evaluated the four papers, co-authored by Blakemore that he himself cited in a May 1987 defense of his vision deprivation experiments.[5] First, we examined the clinical relevance of the four papers. Then, we reviewed citations to these works in order to determine whether clinicians found Blakemore's research valuable. Finally, we considered this research's applicability to the leading clinical issues in the management of strabismus and amblyopia.

Part 1: Review of Four of Blakemore's Papers

1) Blakemore C, van Sluyters RC. "Reversal of the physiological effects of monocular deprivation in kittens."[6]

Blakemore and van Sluyters studied the effect of suturing one eye in kittens on the sensitivity of visual cortex neurons. The main findings were a) "suturing the lids of one eye until 5 weeks of age leaves virtually every neurone in the kitten's visual cortex entirely dominated by the other eye," b) "reverse suturing at 5 weeks caused a complete switch in ocular dominance," and c) "between 5 weeks and 4 months of age, there is a period of declining sensitivity to both the effects of an initial period of monocular deprivation and the reversal of those effects by reverse suturing."[6]

a) Long before visual deprivation experiments on animals began in the early 1960s, it was known that occlusion of an eye in children, for example by cataract or corneal opacity, causes amblyopia.[7-11] The later animal experiments merely accorded with clinical studies. For example, Peter wrote in 1932, "Any interference with the clarity of the media in one eye will produce a definite delay in the completion of the development (which) may be . . . beyond the time when development is possible."[7] Blakemore and van Sluyters, as well as many other investigators, suggested that changes in ocular dominance due to occlusion of an eye during an early "critical period" accounted for amblyopia. However, there is good reason to doubt the validity of these findings for human amblyopia. It is well known that the vision of an amblyopic eye often improves at any age, if the patient is forced to use that eye.[12] For example, total therapeutic occlusion of the "good" eye in late childhood will improve the vision of the amblyopic eye, but this improvement is lost when occlusion of the good eye ceases. Similarly, an elderly patient who is blinded in the "good" eye, e.g., by cataract, will often experience substantially improved vision in a severely amblyopic eye. Removal of the cataract from the "good" eye will result in deterioration of vision in the amblyopic eye. Thus, Blakemore and van Sluyters' studies of cortical dominance in experimental animals may reflect artifacts of the extreme visual disability tested in the laboratory. The relevance of their research to normal or abnormal human physiology is questionable.

b) Blakemore and van Sluyters showed that kittens, like humans, have a period of visual system plasticity. While there is evidence that excessive therapeutic patching of a human patient's eye (to treat amblyopia) reverses the eye that develops amblyopia,[13] the extreme reverse patching in this experiment has no apparent clinical correlate. Thus, there are no clinical data to confirm or contradict Blakemore and van Sluyters' findings. Nevertheless, common sense tells us that extreme reverse patching will reverse the eye that becomes amblyopic. It was well known prior to this experiment 1) that cessation of "occlusion" of an eye (e.g., removal of a cataract) during the critical period will improve the vision of the amblyopic eye and also 2) that excessive occlusion during the critical period can cause amblyopia. Blakemore and van Sluyters merely did the former to one eye and the latter to the other eye.

While this research's clinical relevance is questionable, Blakemore and van Sluyters made observations about ocular dominance associated with visual deprivation which may be of "basic science" interest. This area of inquiry, involving scores of investigators worldwide, was inspired by the Nobel Prize winning work of Hubel and Wiesel.[14] Such research has fascinated many people, but its clinical value has been challenged.[15] Studies designed to elucidate amblyopia's pathology at the cellular level do not necessarily advance our understanding of the conditions that cause amblyopia, our ability to treat amblyopia, or our ability to determine the prognosis for individual amblyopic patients (see section 3).

c) Blakemore and van Sluyters described a critical period for the development of amblyopia in kittens. Human children, too, have a critical period. However, the age at which visual deprivation causes amblyopia is species specific. Thus, full characterization of the critical period in cats or any other nonhuman species provides no useful information about the critical period for children. In fact, the animal research can be misleading. Vaegan and Taylor have noted, "Children appear to have a critical period which continues for longer than expected from animal models."[16] This critical period is being characterized by ongoing clinical investigation. For example, clinicians are assessing the amblyopia that develops from congenital cataracts removed at different times in childhood.

Is eyelid suturing analogous to other forms of amblyopia? The relevance of sutured eyelids to congenital cataracts in children is questionable. Crawford and Marc have noted, "It is not clear whether the result of eyelid suturing can be attributed solely to form deprivation or to reduced light input to the eye."[17] Metz has remarked that eyelid suturing is very different from occlusion amblyopia, and he has expressed concern that the experimental data may be misinterpretted to indicate that patching amblyopes causes more harm than good.[17a]

2) Blakemore C, van Sluyters RC. "Experimental analysis of amblyopia and strabismus"[18]

This paper is largely a review of animal "models" of amblyopia due to occlusion and to strabismus. As in the case of occlusive amblyopia, strabismic amblyopia was described in human patients long before the animal models were used.[19] In this paper, Blakemore and van Sluyters note that animals raised in a visual environment artificially restricted to striped lines retained binocular innervation of cortical cells. Presumably, the animals therefore possessed binocular vision, even if the eyes were strabismic.

Although Blakemore and van Sluyters suggest that therapy involving striped lines to stimulate the cortical cells may someday contribute to a therapy for strabismic patients, to our knowledge, no treatment of this kind is currently in use. Indeed, Blakemore has acknowledged, "If one keeps up the binocular stimulation of the cortex while not correcting the strabismus, then one may generate another problem -- a condition far worse than amblyopia, namely the diplopia (double vision) which should result."[18]

3) Eggers HM, Blakemore C. "Physiological basis of anisometropic amblyopia"[20]

Long before animal research on anisometropia began, clinicians knew that anisometropia can cause amblyopia.[21-23] In order to produce anisometropia in kittens, Eggers and Blakemore fitted them with glasses with one strong minus lens. Not surprisingly, the researchers found changes in ocular dominance in the cortex similar to, but not as complete as, those resulting from monocular occlusion. It is not certain if these data can be applied to human children. First, unlike the experimental kittens, nearly all children with clinically significant anisometropia have similar focusing power of the eyes. Their anisometropia results from differences in the *size* of the eyes. The larger eye generally has thinned tissues, which can adversely affect vision. The animal model does not parallel this problem. Second, the feline visual system is a poor analogue to the human one.[24-27] Von Noorden has noted:

> Amblyopia has now been produced successfully in models of various species, but data from cats, squirrels, and dogs cannot be applied automatically to man. There are differences in the anatomic and functional organization of the visual system of cats and primates . . . Human amblyopia involves primarily foveal vision rather than peripheral vision, and a cat has no fovea.[28]

4) Swindale NV, Vital-Durand F, Blakemore C. "Recovery from monocular deprivation in the monkey"[29]

Swindale, Vital-Durand, and Blakemore studied the effects of monocular deprivation on ocular dominance in a particular cortical layer of the *Erythrocebus patas* (Old World) monkey's brain. In this highly popular area of inquiry, researchers describe, in detail, the effect of visual deprivation on specific cortical areas. This research assists in the "mapping" of the visual system's neural pathways. The practical applications of such findings, however, appear to be nil. For example, assuming that the data derived from other animals can be extrapolated to humans, this line of research demonstrated that areas 2, 3, and 5 of each lateral geniculate body receive neurons from the eye on the same side, and that areas 1, 4, and 6 receive neurons from the eye on the opposite side. Although this information is generally taught to students of ophthalmology,[30] it has not, to our knowledge, changed our understanding or treatment of any eye disorder. Furthermore, some of this information can be safely and non-invasively obtained from human subjects with PET scans,[31-33] CAT scans,[34] and autopsy studies.[35]

This research should be considered "basic science," in that it attempts to add to our basic knowledge of the visual system. It is important to note, however, that Blakemore and van Sluyters did *not* study vision *per se*. They recorded electric firing of neurons, which is not the same as perception of visual images. The firing of neurons is certainly related to vision, but the nature of this relationship is not known.

Part 2: *Science Citation Index* Review

The *Science Citation Index*, through 1991, lists 376 citations to the four papers discussed above. We were able to obtain and review all but 12 of these articles. Several of the articles cited more than one of the four papers written by Blakemore and colleagues. In order to assess the clinical impact of the research of Blakemore and associates, we evaluated all 35 articles that involved research with human subjects. While one would expect animal researchers to focus on the laboratory research implications of the cited studies, investigators working with human subjects are more likely to accurately assess the laboratory's contributions to the understanding of human anatomy, physiology, and pathology. Review articles were omitted because it was not possible to determine whether the authors' primary interests were in laboratory science or clinical investigation. While most references to the four papers by Blakemore and associates are by fellow animal researchers, many clinical investigators have also cited them. Few clinical researchers, however, have credited Blakemore and colleagues with important contributions.

In their citations, many clinical scientists note that Blakemore and colleagues found a critical period for occlusion amblyopia[36-45] and for anisometropic amblyopia.[46-49] One report mentions that reverse patching can reverse the eye that develops amblyopia,[50] two papers note that occlusion causes amblyopia,[45,51] and two papers state only that amblyopia has been studied in animals.[52,53] As was discussed above, before the work by Blakemore and associates, it was already well known that human children have a critical period for the development of amblyopia. Indeed, some of the clinical researchers citing Blakemore and colleagues also cite human clinical reports on amblyopia's critical period that were published before 1974 (the date of the earliest paper discussed above).[36,38,39,43,44,49] Two authors add that, while the critical period has been described in certain laboratory animals, more human clinical research is needed to determine the critical period for humans.[39,41] Campbell et al. have written:

> The time course of these improvements and the age at which they occur (in children) do not tally in any simple manner with the numerous studies of the 'critical period' for visual deprivation in cats and monkeys. It is very unlikely that the amblyopes that we have studied have actually *lost* neurones which

> subsequently regenerate with treatment. It seems more probable, in the light of the treatment time course, that neurones in amblyopia have reduced function.[37]

Some papers discussed the specific findings of cortical neuron recordings. Four of these mention reversal of cortical dominance patterns with reverse patching[42,44,54,55]; one also comments on the finding that reverse patching reduces the number of binocularly driven cells.[44] Both points were discussed above. This information may be of intellectual interest, but its clinical relevance is doubtful.

Several papers cite the work of Eggers and Blakemore[20] for demonstrating that, in anisometropic amblyopia, most cortical neurons are monocularly driven[56-58] and that those cortical cells that respond to the blurred eye[57-69] show decreased contrast sensitivity. The first point is an electrophysiological representation of a phenomenon that can easily be demonstrated in people. Loss of binocular vision can be seen and tested in amblyopes. The questionable value of this electrophysiological research has been discussed above. The second point is not directly applicable to contrast sensitivity as a measure of visual acuity. Eggers and Blakemore did not study *visual* contrast sensitivity, but the contrast sensitivity of cortical neurons as determined by their firing rates. The correlation between their electrophysiological studies and vision is not known. Interestingly, tests of visual acuity as measured by contrast sensitivity were done with human patients prior to Eggers and Blakemore's work. One clinical report[64] cites three papers on contrast sensitivity in human amblyopes that precede Eggers and Blakemore's 1978 study.

Two papers warrant further discussion. Thomas[70] cited Blakemore and van Sluyters[6] in support of a theory that amblyopia involves larger receptor fields. At present, this speculation can be neither confirmed nor refuted. Current technology does not permit microelectrode studies of cortical receptive fields in humans.

Only one clinical paper explicitly endorses the animal model.[43] Jastrzebski et al. have written:

> Examination of the effects of compromised visual experience on the young visual system in animals has been useful as a probe into its structure, function, and development. The importance of the animal model to the clinician arises from a need for some physiological basis for the cause, diagnosis, therapy, and prognosis of stimulus deprivation amblyopia. . . . The benefit of reverse deprivation in improving the amblyopic eye is apparent both from the animal data and clinical practice. It is also clear that reverse deprivation must take place during a sensitive period.[43]

The first sentence notes that the animal research has provided information on neuroanatomy, visual system development, and visual electrophysiology. The clinical value of this research, to date, has been questionable. The second sentence, a broad endorsement of animal research, provides no details of how the animal model may be used to address these clinically important issues. The last two sentences discuss the existence of the critical period for the development and for the reversal of amblyopia in both people and animals. Interestingly, one of the many citations used in support of this point was a clinical study from 1959.

Few clinicians credit the animal research with important contributions. Indeed, Hess et al. have noted that the relevance of the animal research to humans remains unclear:

> It is obviously much more difficult and hazardous to compare the present psychophysical findings on pattern deprived humans with neurophysiological data from pattern deprived animals. This difficulty in relating single cell responses and psychophysics is further clouded by the conflicting nature of the neurophysiological findings as to the exact physiological consequences of, and structures involved in, monocular pattern deprivation in animals.[51]

Part 3: Relevance of the Research to Clinically Important Issues

It does not appear that visual deprivation experiments, despite their widespread use, have assisted the prevention or treatment of any human patients. While it is not possible to predict the future with certainty, the likelihood of benefit to humans can be assessed by evaluating the relevance of the animal research to the leading clinical questions that concern ophthalmologists.

1) What are the critical periods for the different types of amblyopia (e.g., occlusive, strabismic, anisometropic) in children? The answers would help ophthalmologists determine when to attempt surgical correction of the underlying defect(s). The age at which human children are at risk for the development of amblyopia depends on the time course of the human ocular system's development. Since different species have different critical periods, the human critical period can be determined only by studies and observations of human children. The critical periods of other animals may be determined in the laboratory, but such information cannot be extrapolated to humans. Amblyopia's development from vision deprivation has been common knowledge for decades, and characterization of the human critical period began long before the animal experiments. In 1921, Juler commented on traumatic cataracts in children, "There is a striking line of difference between the final vision results depending on the age at which the injury occurred."[71]

Having performed extensive research on visual deprivation in animals, von Noorden has concluded:

> This period of susceptibility of the visual system to unilateral visual deprivation, whatever the cause, has been well defined in kittens and monkeys but not in children. Such information is needed, however, to determine how soon to operate on a congenital cataract or traumatic cataract during childhood, the age at which

> to consider a corneal transplant for a congenital or acquired corneal opacity, or when to correct anisometropia to preserve sight in an eye that otherwise will become irreversibly amblyopic. . . . The only information available at this time is that gleaned from retrospective analysis of individual cases.[72]

2) What is the effect of amblyopic conditions on binocular vision and stereovision? It is difficult to test binocular vision in laboratory animals. The inability of animals to articulate their perceptions is a barrier to assessing small changes in visual function. While clinicians have the same problem with infants, small children can describe what they see, enhancing the informative value of visual tests. Blakemore and van Sluyters have acknowledged, "Our tests of behavioral function are extremely crude by the standards that are applied to humans, and they would probably only reveal a deficit so great that it would be regarded in the human as some form of blindness, not amblyopia."[18]

3) When should we operate to straighten the eyes in strabismic children? This complicated issue has generated much debate among ophthalmologists. Von Noorden has addressed this issue in the 1987 Jackson Memorial Lecture. Discussing essential esotropia, a category that includes the majority of strabismus cases in children, he has noted that an understanding of the condition's etiology is critical. Some investigators believe that the strabismus is due to a congenitally defective fusional mechanism; consequently the children do not have the normal ability to fuse the images of the two eyes. Others maintain that a defect in the neuronal innervation of the muscles causes misalignment of the eyes. The former theory would favor conservative treatment, while the latter theory would suggest that early surgery may be warranted to improve vision, even though the risks of anaesthesia are greater for younger infants. Von Noorden has observed:

> These two opposing views have far-reaching therapeutic implications. If esotropia is caused by an inborn defect of the fusion faculty, no treatment, no matter how early in life, will restore normalcy. If, on the other hand, no such defect exists, a cure could be accomplished by aligning the eyes as early as possible.[72]

He continues:

> We must ask whether animal experiments have helped us to better understand the pathophysiology of essential infantile esotropia. Such experiments are cited by proponents of early surgery as they allegedly show an irreversible deterioration of binocular pathways in cats and monkeys with strabismus during infancy. . . . However . . . there is no evidence from animal research that binocular functions other than stereopsis, such as sensory and motor fusion, are similarly affected by abnormal visual experience early in life. There is currently no animal model for essential infantile esotropia.[72]

Strabismus is created in experimental animals by surgical manipulation of muscles. This is different from either of the two mechanisms proposed for the development of human essential esotropia, i.e., congenital deficiency of innate fusion or abnormal innervation of the eye muscles. Artificially induced misalignment of the eyes is not the same as spontaneous strabismus in children; the etiology of human strabismus cannot be determined by studies with laboratory animals.

4) What is the nature of amblyopia? Answers to this question may assist the management of this condition. Even if data from electrophysiological research with animals were known to be applicable to human amblyopia, such research does not address the basic visual disturbances that characterize amblyopia. To provide the necessary information, studies often rely on effective communication between the subject and the examiner. For example, there is evidence based on subtle contrast sensitivity testing in humans that there are two kinds of amblyopia due to strabismus.[73] Similarly, human studies of anomalous retinal correspondence (ARC) have yielded considerable insight into binocular vision. (It is difficult, if not impossible, to assess ARC from animal electrophysiologic studies.) ARC is an adaptation to strabismus, in which the cortical input from the deviating eye is somehow "re-programmed" by the brain to permit both eyes to see the same object (binocular vision.) A greater understanding of the basis of ARC may help elucidate the mechanism of cortical plasticity in humans. Of more direct clinical relevance, however, is the fact that ARC can represent a formidable obstacle to proper alignment of the eyes and recovery of normal binocular vision after strabismus surgery. It is unclear whether ARC occurs in nonhuman animals because behavioral tests are too crude to evaluate this brain adaptation. To date, ARC has not been found in experimental animals.[74] Perhaps other animals possess the potential for ARC, but we cannot study ARC in the laboratory due to our difficulty in communicating with the animals.

Finally, two valuable observations of visual function in amblyopia could have been derived only from human clinical investigation. Amblyopes can read smaller letters on a vision chart if the letters are isolated than if they are one of a series or field of letters. This is known as "crowding phenomenon."[75] Also, the amblyopic eye can see as well, or almost as well, as the normal eye under conditions of reduced illumination.[76] These observations, which are much easier to evaluate with human subjects, offer insights into the nature of amblyopia that electrophysiological testing cannot address.

Conclusions

Blakemore and colleagues have studied various forms of visual disability in laboratory animals. In extensive review of the literature, we found no evidence that our understanding amblyopia's causes or treatments have improved as a consequence of this research. Furthermore, because experimental models of amblyopia cannot address the issues of critical importance to practicing clinicians these models' future benefit to human patients is doubtful. It is unlikely that the public would wish scarce financial resources to be allocated to such research for the sake of "pure knowledge." Unfortunately, Blakemore has defended his work on the grounds that it is important to human patients.[1] The claim appears to lack factual support.

Acknowledgement
We would like to thank Gill Langley, Ph.D. for invaluable research and editorial assistance.

References

1. Langley G. *Blinded by science: The facts about sight deprivation experiments on animals.* Animal Aid, 1987.
2. Sharpe R. *The Cruel Deception.* Wellingborough, Thorsons Publishers, 1988.
3. Buyukmihci NC. Response to Dr. Blakemore's assertion that work involving nonhuman animals has led to significantly greater understanding and treatment of amblyopia. *Perspec An Res* 1989;1:57-62.
4. Blakemore C. Misguided thinking on animals. *Nature* 1989;339:414.
5. Blakemore C. *A reply to criticism of experiments involving visual deprivation.* May 1987.
6. Blakemore C, van Sluyters RC. Reversal of the physiological effects of monocular deprivation in kittens: further evidence for a sensitive period. *J Physiol* 1974;237:195-216.
7. Peter LC. Symposium on the treatment of non-paralytic squint. *Trans Ophth Soc UK* 1932;52:325-380.
8. Braendstrup P. Amblyopia ex anopsia in infantile cataract. *Acta Ophthalmol Kbh* 1944;22:52-71.
9. Juler F. Amblyopia from disuse: Visual acuity after traumatic cataract in children. *Trans Ophthal Soc UK* 1921:41;129.
10. Abraham SV. A tribute to Claude Worth. *Ann Ophthalmol* 1972;4:171-175.
11. Cibis L. Fifth annual Richard G. Scobee Memorial Lecture: History of amblyopia and its treatment. *Am Orthop J* 1975;2:193-225.
12. Vereecken EP, Brabant P. Prognosis for vision in amblyopia after the loss of the good eye. *Arch Ophthalmol* 1984;102:220-224.
13. Awaya A, Miyaki Y, Imaizumi Y, Shinose Y, Kanda T, Komoru K. Amblyopia in man, suggestive of stimulus deprivation amblyopia. *Jpn J Ophthalmol* 1973;17:69-82.
14. Hubel DH, Wiesel TN. Binocular interaction in striate cortex of kittens reared with artificial squint. *J Neurophysiol* 1965;28:1041-1059.
15. Drewett R, Kani W. Animal experimentation in the behavioral sciences. In, Sperlinger D (ed): *Animals in Research.* New York, Wiley, 1981, pp 175-201.
16. Vaegan, Taylor D. Critical period for deprivation amblyopia in children. *Trans Ophth Soc* 1979;99:432-441.
17. Crawford MLJ, Marc RE. Light transmission of cat and monkey eyelids. *Vision Res* 1976;16:323-324.
17a. Metz HS. Letter to the editor. *Invest Ophth Vis Sci* 1985;26:249.
18. Blakemore C, van Sluyters RC. Experimental analysis of amblyopia and strabismus. *Brit J*

Ophthal 1974;58:176-182.
19. Chavasse B. Symposium on non-paralytic squint; comment. *Trans Ophthal Soc UK* 1932;52:348-352.
20. Eggers HM, Blakemore C. Physiological basis of anisometropic amblyopia. *Science* 1978;201:264-267.
21. Copps LA. Vision in anisometropia. *Am J Ophthalmol* 1944;23:641-644.
22. Jampolsky A, Flom BC, Weymouth F, Moses LE. Unequal corrected visual acuity as related to anisometropia. *Arch Ophthalmol* 1955;54:893-905.
23. Philips CI. Strabismus, anisometropia, and amblyopia. *Brit J Ophthalmol* 1959;43:449-460.
24. Headon MP, Sloper JJ, Hiorns RW, Powell TPS. Sizes of neurons in the primate lateral geniculate nucleus during normal development. *Dev Brain Res* 1985;18:51-56.
25. Lewis TL, Maurer D, Brent HP. Optokinetic nystagmus in normal and visually deprived children: Implications for cortical development. *Can J Psychol* 1989;43:121-140.
26. Shapley R, Perry VH. Cat and monkey retinal ganglion cells and their visual functional roles. *Trends Neurosci* 1986;9:227-235.
27. Marg E. Printice Memorial Lecture: Is the animal model for stimulus deprivation amblyopia in children valid or useful? *Am J Optomet Physiol Optics* 1982;59:451-464.
28. von Noorden GK. Application of basic research data to clinical amblyopia. *Ophthalmology* 1978;85:496-504.
29. Swindale NV, Vital-Durand F, Blakemore C. Recovery from monocular deprivation in the monkey. III. Reversal of anatomical effects in the cortex. *Proc R Soc Lond B* 1981;213:435-450.
30. American Academy of Ophthalmology. *Basic and Clinical Science Course, Section 5: Neuro-ophthalmology*. San Francisco, American Academy of Ophthalmology, 1988, p 48.
31. Fox PT, Mintun MA, Raichle ME, Miezin FM, Allman JM, Van Essen DC. Mapping human visual cortex with positron emission tomography. *Nature* 1986;323:806-809.
32. Kushner MJ, Rosenquist A, Alavi A, et al. Cerebral metabolism and patterned visual stimulation: A positron emission tomographic study of the human visual cortex. *Neurology* 1988;38:89-95.
33. Demer JL, von Noorden GK, Volkow ND, Gould KL. Imaging of cerebral blood flow and metabolism in amblyopia by positron emission tomography. *Am J Ophthalmol* 1988;105:337-347.
34. McAuley DL, Ross Russell RW. Correlation of CAT scan and visual field defects in vascular lesions of the posterior visual pathways. *J Neurol Neurosurg Psychiat* 1979;42:298-311.
35. von Noorden GK, Crawford MLJ, Levacy RA. The lateral geniculate nucleus in human anisometropic amblyopia. *Invest Ophthalmol Vis Sci* 1983;24:788-790.
36. Glass JD, Crowder JV, Kennerdell JS, Merikangus JR. Visually evoked potentials from occipital and precentral cortex in visually deprived humans. *Electroencephalography Clin Neurophysiol* 1977;43:207-217.
37. Campbell FW, Hess RF, Watson PG, Banks R. Preliminary results of a physiologically based treatment of amblyopia. *Brit J Ophthalmol* 1978;62:748-755.
38. Dunlop P, Dunlop D. Infant strabismus: A 25-year review of 750 cases. *Med J Australia* 1979;1:111-113.
39. Ingram RM. Amblyopia: The need for a new approach? *Brit J Ophthalmol* 1979;63:236-237.
40. Arden GB, Barnard WM. Effect of occlusion on the visual evoked response in amblyopia. *Trans Ophthal Soc UK* 1979;99:419-426.
41. Rogers GL, Tishler CL, Tsori BH, Hertle RW, Gellows RR. Visual acuities in infants with congenital cataracts operated on prior to 6 months of age. *Arch Ophthalmol* 1981;99:999-1003.
42. Prakash P, Grover AK, Khosla PK, Gahlot DK. Ocular motility in alternating squints: An

electro-oculographic study. *Brit J Ophthalmol* 1982;66:258-263.

43. Jastrzebski GB, Hoyt CS, Marg E. Stimulus deprivation amblyopia in children: sensitivity, plasticity, and elasticity (SPE). *Arch Ophthalmol* 1984;102:1030-1034.
44. Billson FA, Fitzgerald BA, Provis JM. Visual deprivation in infancy and childhood: Clinical aspects. *Austral New Zeal J Ophthalmol* 1985;13:279-286.
45. Awaya S, Sugawara M, Miyake S, Isomura Y. Form vision amblyopia and the result of its treatment -- with special reference to the critical period. *Jpn J Ophthalmol* 1980;24:241-250.
46. Barris MC, Dawson WW, Trick LR. LASCER bode plots for normal, amblyopic, and stereoanomalous observers. *Doc Ophthalmol* 1981;51:347-363.
47. Levi DM, Manny RE. The pathophysiology of amblyopia: Electrophysiological studies. *Ann NY Acad Sci* 1982;388:243-263.
48. Persson HE, Wanger P. Pattern-reversal electroretinograms in squint amblyopia, artificial anisometropia and simulated eccentric fixation. *Acta Ophthalmol* 1982;60:123-132.
49. Howland HC, Sayles N. A photorefractive characterization of focusing ability of infants and young children. *Invest Ophthalmol Vis Sci* 1987;28:1005-1015.
50. Awaya S, Sugawara M, Miyake S. Observations in patients with occlusion amblyopia. *Trans Ophthal Soc UK* 1979;99:447-454.
51. Hess RF, France TD, Tulunay-Keesey U. Residual vision in humans who have been monocularly deprived of pattern stimulation in early life. *Exp Brain Res* 1981;44:295-311.
52. Hess RF, Baker CL. Assessment of retinal function in severely amblyopic individuals. *Vision Res* 1984;24:1367-1376.
53. Hess RF, Pointer JS. Differences in the neural basis of human amblyopia: The distribution of the anomaly accross the visual field. *Vision Res* 1984;25:1577-1594.
54. Loshin DS, Levi DM. Suprathreshold contrast perception in functional amblyopia. *Doc Ophthalmol* 1983;55:213-236.
55. Kani W. Stereopsis and spatial perception in amblyopes and uncorrected ametropes. *Brit J Ophthalmol* 1978;62:756-762.
56. Levi DM, Harwerth RS, Smith EL. Binocular interactions in normal and anomalous binocular vision. *Doc Ophthalmol* 1980;49:303-324.
57. Bradley A, Freeman RD. Contrast sensitivity in anisometropic amblyopia. *Invest Ophthalmol Vis Sci* 1981;21:467-476.
58. Mohn G, Hof-van Duin J. On the relation of stereoacuity to interocular transfer of the motion and the tilt aftereffects. *Vision Res* 1983;23:1087-1096.
59. Hess RF, Campbell FW, Zimmern R. Differences in the neural basis of human amblyopias: The effect of mean luminance. *Vision Res* 1980;20:295-305.
60. Hess RF, Burr DC, Campbell FW. A preliminary investigation of neural function and dysfunction in amblyopia - III: Co-operative activity of amblyopic channels. *Vision Res* 1980;20:757-760.
61. Levi DM, Harwerth RS, Pass AF, Venverloh J. Edge sensitivity mechanisms in humans with abnormal visual experience. *Exp Brain Res* 1981;43:270-280.
62. Selby SA, Woodhouse JM. The spatial frequency dependence of interocular transfer in amblyopia. *Vision Res* 1981;21:1401-1408.
63. Sireteanu R, Fronius M. Naso-temporal asymmetries in human amblyopia: Consequences of long-term interocular suppression. *Vision Res* 1981;21:1055-1064.
64. Sjostrand J. Contrast sensitivity in children with strabismic and anisometropic amblyopia. A study of the effect of treatment. *Acta Ophthalmol* 1981;59:25-34.
65. Hess RF. Contrast-coding in amblyopia II. On the physiological basis of contrast recruitment. *Proc Roy Soc B* 1983;217:331-340.
66. Katz LM, Levi DM, Bedell HE. Central and peripheral contrast sensitivity in amblyopia with varying field size. *Doc Ophthalmol* 1985;58:351-373.

67. Levi DM, Klein SA, Yap YL. Positional uncertainty in peripheral and amblyopic vision. *Vision Res* 1987;27:581-597.
68. Barbeito R, Bedell HE, Flom MC, Simpson TL. Effects of luminance on the visual acuity of strabismic and anisometropic amblyopes and optically blurred animals. *Vision Res* 1987;27:1543-1549.
69. Levi DM, Klein SA. Equivalent intrinsic blur in amblyopia. *Vision Res* 1990;30:1995-2022.
70. Thomas J. Normal and amblyopic contrast sensitivity functions in central and peripheral retinas. *Invest Ophthalmol Vis Sci* 1978;17:746-753.
71. Juler F. Amblyopia from disease. Visual acuity after traumatic cataract in children. *Trans Ophthal Soc UK* 1921;41:129-138.
72. von Noorden GK. A reassessment of infantile esotropia. XLIV Edward Jackson Memorial Lecture. *Am J Ophthal* 1988;105:1-10.
73. Hess RF, Howell ER. The threshold contrast sensitivity function in strabismic amblyopia: Evidence for a two type classification. *Vision Res* 1977;17:1049-1055.
74. Lang J. Anomalous retinal correspondence update. *Graefe's Arch Ophthalmol* 1988;226:137-140.
75. von Noorden GK. *Atlas of Strabismus*, 4th Ed. London, CV Mosby, 1983.
76. von Noorden GK, Burian HM. Visual acuity in normal and amblyopic patients under reduced illumination. *Arch Ophthalmol* 1959;61:533-535.

Scientific Problems with Animal Models

Stephen R. Kaufman

Historian and philosopher of science Thomas Kuhn notes that every scientific age has its "paradigms," theories nearly universally regarded as true that form the framework for ongoing scientific investigations.[1] Paradigms are rarely challenged until overwhelming contradictory evidence forces their revision or rejection. A currently dominant paradigm is that animal "models" are necessary for medical progress.[2-4] For most members of the current scientific establishment, the issue is not whether animal models should be used but which models are most useful. However, critics of animal models argue that they are inherently flawed[5-7] and point out the frequency with which animal models provide misleading information.[8-12]

All species differ; animal-model conditions never *exactly* mimic human ones. Animal models are only *analogues* of human conditions because they share certain characteristics. Philosophers Hugh LaFollette and Niall Shanks observe that animal models are used primarily for two functions--to predict human responses to stimuli (such as infectious, traumatic, or toxic conditions and therapeutic drugs or devices) and to offer new ways of conceptualizing human anatomy, physiology, or pathology. Researchers who use animal models employ the following reasoning: a given animal model resembles an analogous human condition in some of its features (say, A, B, and C); therefore, it is reasonable to proceed as if an additional feature (D) found in the animal model--for example, a physiological function or a drug response--can be expected to be a feature of the human condition as well. As LaFollette and Shanks point out, this assertion is logical only if feature D is *causally* related to A, B, and C--in both the animal model and the human condition. That is, A, B, and C must be *causal factors* of feature D. The following reasoning illustrates a failure to recognize the importance of causal relationships:

> Two dogs bark, love bones, and wag their tails when their human companions arrive home; because the two dogs are similar in these respects, they can also be expected to be of the same breed. If we know the first dog's breed, we can reliably predict the second's.

Breed, however, is not causally related to the three features that the two dogs are already known to share. If we know a dog's breed and we *also* know that a second dog has the same parents as the first, then we can reliably predict the second dog's breed--even if the two dogs differ in many other respects, such as coat color or temperament.

LaFollette and Shanks distinguish between weak and strong models. Strong animal models are identical to the analogous human features in *all* causally relevant respects, and research using such models can be confidently applied to humans. Although many animal research advocates assert that animal models faithfully reproduce human conditions, LaFollette and Shanks argue that most animal models are weak models of little direct applicability to humans. Nevertheless, LaFollette and Shanks do not reject animal research's value. They maintain that animal models may be helpful but are probably not *necessary* for medical progress.[5]

In public, animal research proponents often suggest that weak causal models are in fact strong. For example, the Stanford Committee on Ethics states, "Cancer kills humans and animals alike."[13] At any but the most simplistic level, the comparison immediately begins to break down. For example, malignancies that are experimentally induced in nonhuman animals and malignancies that occur spontaneously in humans significantly differ in their *causes*.[14-16] Other important differences include the greater virulence of most experimental cancer strains and differing mechanisms of tumor growth and metastasis. Even nonhuman cancers that apparently share many characteristics with human cancers make unreliable research models, since human and nonhuman cancers inevitably differ in *some* relevant causal factors. Viewed in this light, an animal model such as the mouse-leukemia model is a poor means of attempting to identify potential anti-cancer drugs, and this model has, in fact, proved grossly inadequate.[17]

Even if a disease's main causal factors were well understood--and were alike--in both humans and other animals, animal models would still be undermined by *systemic* differences between animal models and human conditions. Because of evolutionary divergence, species show differences in virtually every aspect of organ and tissue function. All organ subsystems interact, so every physiological difference between a given "laboratory"-animal species and the human species necessarily affect every causal factor. Consequently, *all* tissues of an animal model will tend to react to an experimental manipulation differently from a supposedly analogous human condition. Animal models of human conditions tend to provide only the most obvious and general information, such as that cancers kill; in order for them to provide reliable and specific information, the model and the human condition must have identical causal factors and have no significant systemic differences that affect these causal factors. This is impossible, since there are always differences in causal factors between the model and the human condition and because systemic differences are an inevitable consequence of evolutionary divergence.

In theory, then, animal modeling is unreliable in predicting human responses to stimuli; and it has proved so in practice. Animal tests of acute lethal toxicity,[18] eye irritancy,[19-21] skin irritancy,[22-24] teratogenesis (birth defects),[25-27] and carcinogenesis[28,29] have generally provided inconsistent results and failed to correspond to human experience. R. Heywood has estimated that only about 5-25% of toxic effects found in animal experiments occur in humans.[30] Of course, animal models can serve as strong models when researchers attempt to predict gross toxicological effects, such as the ability of strong acids to burn the eye's surface; however, such effects could readily be predicted from the most rudimentary knowledge of chemistry. Most animal tests are supposedly intended to identify *subtle* effects, and they perform poorly in this regard.

Animal tests have also proved inadequate as a means of identifying potentially useful drugs. U.S. law requires that drugs be found effective and safe in animal testing before they are tested on humans. This law fails to reflect animal tests' poor predictive value: Ronald Hansen found that only about 12% of drugs that passed Phase I animal tests and entered human testing reached the market;[31] earlier, Samuel Irwin had found that only 2.3% of drugs selected for clinical trial were eventually marketed.[32] Most new drugs are similar to existing drugs, and so their clinical effect can be at least partially predicted based on structural analogy. Also, modern biochemical methods can help characterize specific drug-receptor interactions, and these interactions can suggest specific drug effects. Therefore, it is debatable whether animal tests help identify which drugs are most suitable for human clinical trials (the critical step in determining *human* safety and efficacy).

In addition to having failed to accurately predict drugs' efficacy and toxic side-effects, animal tests have, no doubt, prompted researchers to abandon numerous drugs and therapies that proved ineffective or toxic in nonhuman animals but would have benefitted humans. It is impossible to determine how many valuable therapies were discarded on the basis of misleading animal studies.

Are animal models worthless, then? Although causal dissimilarities and systemic differences *undermine* animal models, they are not *necessarily* useless. For example, animal data need not accord perfectly with human data to be relevant. For example an animal test that correctly identified carcinogens 90% of the time could help formulate reasonable public health guidelines. However, as noted above, most animal tests do not accurately identify subtle toxic effects. Therefore, animal toxicity data may be valuable in theory, but in practice it is generally inconsistent and misleading.

Although most animal models are weak models, certain strong ones can reliably predict gross toxicological effects. For example canaries were once used to test for carbon monoxide in coal mines because canaries are much more sensitive to this toxic gas than humans are. Although animal models cannot reliably elucidate mechanisms of disease induction and spread in humans, they have, in the past, afforded strong models for research on the organisms themselves. To illustrate, rats infected with the syphilis spirochete yield little insight into human syphilis infection. Nevertheless, Erhlich discovered arsenobenzol as a treatment for syphilis by infecting rats with the spirochete and then trying different compounds for possible anti-syphilis effect. In Ehrlich's studies, rats served primarily as reservoirs to harbor the organism, facilitating research on the *organism itself.* Today, *in vitro* cultures have replaced animals as mere reservoirs for almost all infectious agents.

Also, animal models may provide information about the species under investigation, because there are generally few major differences in physiological parameters among individuals of the same species. Most animal experimenters, however, claim to address *human* health issues.

Many philosophers of science have distinguished between validating (or disproving) hypotheses and formulating them.[33-35] An animal model cannot be used to test a hypothesis about humans because differences in causal factors between the animal model and the human condition render the animal model invalid as a predictor. The only way to support or disprove a hypothesis about human anatomy, physiology, or pathology is by studying human beings. Animal-model conditions are analogues, and it is impossible to validate or disprove any hypothesis by analogy. Therefore, *logically* animal models cannot directly contribute to medical discovery. Medical historian Brandon Reines maintains that animal models primarily "dramatize" hypotheses about humans without actually validating or disproving them.

Although animal models cannot validate or disprove hypotheses, they may function as *heuristic* devices that *assist* the process of discovery.[5-7] That is, they may suggest different ways of conceptualizing problems and thereby help generate new hypotheses. In this regard *weak* models have potential value. An unexpected finding during animal experimentation (including experimentation that was poorly conducted or that failed to accomplish its original objectives) may lead to an insight.

Such insights, however, can also arise via other research approaches, such as observing human patients, conducting epidemiological studies, performing *in vitro* tests, or engaging in computer or mechanical modeling. Once again, then, animal models do not appear to be *necessary* for medical progress. In fact, medical historian Brandon Reines[36,37] and physician Paul Beeson[38] consider the role of animal models as heuristic aids very limited.

In a review of hepatitis research, Beeson writes: "progress in the understanding and management of human disease must begin, and end, with studies of man."[38] Although much hepatitis research has used animals, Beeson has found that hypotheses about hepatitis have derived from clinical observations, and that clinical studies have been necessary to test their validity.[38]

Reines observes that nearly all hypotheses about human conditions derive from human clinical research.[36,37,39] Animal experimenters, he contends, perform the superfluous and irrelevant function of experimenting with different animal models until they find one that accords with the clinical findings; typically they then claim that their model has "validated" the clinically derived hypothesis. Often, Reines observes, animal modelers highlight confirmatory animal data while discounting animal data that contradict their findings.

Although Beeson doesn't share Reines' conclusion that animal experimentation is largely irrelevant to medical discovery, he agrees that most insights derive from human studies. Beeson writes, "The initial observations of manifestations and courses of human disease must be made in human beings. The important contributions of epidemiology depend on accurate clinical definitions. The occurrence of rare sequels or late manifestations is beyond any feasible approach through experiments on other species."[38] Beeson cites progress in understanding hepatitis, appendicitis, rheumatic fever, typhoid fever, ulcerative colitis, and hyperparathyroidism as representative of most medical progress in having occurred almost exclusively through the study of humans.[38] Nevertheless, like other researchers who have acknowledged the primary importance of clinical investigation yet remain lodged in the animal-model paradigm, Beeson continues to maintain the importance of animal experimentation.[40-45]

The history of polio research illustrates many of animal experimentation's strengths and limitations. Proponents of animal research frequently claim that animal experiments were crucial in controlling polio.[4,46] John R. Paul's review of polio research indicates that animal experimentation facilitated some insights but delayed others.[47]

In the 1800s, polio's clinical presentation and natural history were deduced from bedside observation and post-mortem studies of human victims. Ivar Wickman's detailed epidemiological analyses of two Swedish epidemics in the early 1900s revealed that mild or even subclinical cases contributed to contagious spread of the disease. Most investigators, focusing on polio's life-threatening paralysis, considered polio a central nervous system disease. But Wickman found that polio affects the alimentary tract (throat, stomach, and intestines) and suggested that the gastrointestinal system may be the initial site of infection.[48,49]

By contradicting Wickman's observations, animal data delayed understanding of polio's true pathogenesis and natural history. The first animal model of polio was developed by Simon Flexner, who induced polio-like paralysis in rhesus monkeys after placing infected human tissue into their noses. Convinced that his animal model precisely paralleled the human disease, he concluded that human polio was introduced to the brain via the nose and confined to the central nervous system. For decades, most scientists adhered to this erroneous theory, and this led to misguided therapeutic measures.[47]

While animal studies remained the principal focus of polio research in the United States, Swedish clinical investigators continued to make important contributions. They tested for the presence of polio in tissues of human polio victims and family members by inoculating monkeys with test samples. If a test monkey contracted polio, the sample was determined to be infected. The investigators found that polio carriers could have polio virus present in their throats and intestines up to seven months after exposure. (Here, monkeys were used as bioassays, in which researchers sought a gross effect. Today, few animals are used as bioassays, because more reliable non-animal bioassays exist.)

Meanwhile, Flexner and other animal researchers continued to study rhesus monkeys infected with viruses obtained from other rhesus monkeys. This process selected for more virulent polio strains that tended to infect nervous tissue. Consequently, the animal model increasingly diverged from human polio in pathogenesis and natural history. Systemic differences between humans and rhesus monkeys undermined Flexner's animal model as a causal model of human polio.

In the 1940s researchers found that polio infection in chimpanzees accords more closely to the human disease. Like humans and unlike rhesus monkeys, chimpanzees were found to harbor the polio virus in their alimentary tracts. Researchers were now more willing to accept the clinically derived hypothesis that polio infects the human alimentary tract. But this response merely demonstrates the research establishment's reluctance to accept clinical findings in humans until parallel findings have been produced--however artificially--in the laboratory in another species.

Animal models of polio were not very helpful as causal models, and they significantly delayed development of an effective vaccine. After clinical studies showed that polio virus infects gastrointestinal tissue, decades of experimentation on rhesus monkeys suggested that the virus infects only neural tissue. Vaccine researchers mistakenly believed that polio would only grow in neural tissue, but vaccines derived from these cultures were too dangerous. In 1948, John Enders, Thomas Weller, and Frederick Robbins grew polio on human intestinal tissue, which led to a safe vaccine. Albert Sabin, who developed the Sabin oral polio vaccine, has written, "the work on prevention was long delayed by an erroneous conception of the nature of the human disease based on misleading experimental models of the disease in monkeys."[50]

Nevertheless, animal experiments may have served a heuristic function by inspiring new ways of thinking about polio. For example, studies of TO virus encephalitis in mice revealed that animals infected early in life tend to have a more benign course: after initial exposure to TO virus, mice become immune.[51] According to Paul, this may have helped researchers derive a theory to explain the clinical observation that major epidemics tended to occur in remote areas. Because sparse or isolated populations did not permit an endemic state of polio infection, few children were exposed earlier in life, when the disease tended to have a more benign course. This insight did not *require* animal studies; it could have been derived entirely from clinical investigations, including population studies. The TO virus model illustrates the limited utility of weak models.

Some strong models were also used in the fight against polio. Swedish investigators used monkeys to test for the presence of polio virus in tissue samples; later, researchers used the mouse neutralization test for similar purposes. In addition, monkeys were used in immunological studies that demonstrated multiple distinct viral strains. In these cases, however, researchers merely assessed whether or not the animals became infected under different conditions. Today the absence or presence of a virus in human tissue can be more reliably determined using *in vitro* methods.

In theory and practice, animal models generally fail to reliably predict human responses to stimuli. While some strong animal models exist, most are weak models of human responses to stimuli. Weak animal models may serve as heuristic devices and help to inspire new ways of conceptualizing clinically relevant issues, but they are not indispensable analogues that are directly applicable to humans. As merely heuristic devices, animal models are not necessary for progress in human medicine.

References

1. Kuhn T. *The Structure of Scientific Revolutions*. Chicago, University of Chicago Press, 1969.
2. Bernard C. *An Introduction to the Study of Experimental Medicine*. Paris, Henry Schuman, 1949.
3. American Medical Association. *Use of Animals in Biomedical Research: The Challenge and Response* [White Paper]. Chicago, AMA, 1988.
4. Gay WI (ed). *Health Benefits of Animal Research*. Washington DC, Foundation for Biomedical Research, 1986.
5. LaFollette H, Shanks N. Animal models in biomedical research: Some epistemological worries. *Public Affairs Quarterly* 1992;7(2):113-130.
6. LaFollette H, Shanks N. The intact systems argument: Problems with the standard defense of animal experimentation. *Southern Journal of Philosophy* 1993;31:323-333.
7. LaFollette H, Shanks N. Animal modelling in psychopharmacological contexts. *Behav Br Sci*, Dec. 1993, in press.
8. Peller S. *Quantitative Research in Human Biology and Medicine*. Bristol, John Wright & Sons, 1981.
9. Rowan AN. *Of Mice, Models, & Men: A Critical Evaluation of Animal Research*. Albany, SUNY Press, 1984.
10. Sharpe R. *The Cruel Deception*. Wellingborough, Thorsons Publishers Limited, 1988.
11. Bross ID. *Scientific Fraud vs. Scientific Truth*. Buffalo, Biomedical Metatechnology Press, 1991.
12. Wiebers DO, Adams HP, Whisnant JP. Animal models of stroke: Are they relevant to human disease? *Stroke* 1990;21:1-3.
13. Thomas JA, Hamm TE, Perkins PL, Raffin TA, the Stanford University Medical Center Committee on Ethics. Animal research at Stanford University: Principles, policies, and practices. *N Engl J Med* 1988;318:1630-1632.
14. Kaufman SR, Reines BP, Casele H, Lawson L, Lurie J. Model No. 42: Adenocarcinoma (Rat). *Perspec An Res* 1989;1(suppl):15-26.
15. Bross ID. *Crimes of Official Science: A Casebook*. Buffalo, Biomedical Metatechnology Press, 1987.
16. Reines BP. *Cancer Research on Animals: Impact and Alternatives*. Chicago, National

Anti-Vivisection Society, 1986.

17. Pihl A. UICC Study Group on chemosensitivity testing of human tumors. Problems--applications--future prospects. *Int J Canc* 1986;37:1-5.
18. Zbinden G, Flury-Roversi M. Significance of the LD50 test for toxicological evaluation of chemical substances. *Arch Toxicol* 1981;47:77-99.
19. Weil CS, Scala RA. Study of intra- and interlaboratory variability in the results of rabbit eye and skin irritancy tests. *Toxicol Appl Pharmacol* 1971;19:276-360.
20. Swanson DW. Eye irritancy testing, in Balls M, Riddell RJ, Worden AN (eds). *Animals and Alternatives in Toxicity Testing*. New York, Academic Press, 1983, pp 337-367.
21. Freeberg FE, Hooker DT, Griffith JF. Correlation of animal eye test data with human experience for household products: an update. *J Toxicol-Cutaneous Ocular Toxicol* 1986;5:115-123.
22. Davies RE, Harper KH, Kynoch SR. Inter-species variation in dermal reactivity. J Soc Cosmetic Chemists 1972;23:371-381.
23. Kligman AM. Assessment of mild irritants, in Frost P, Horwitz SN (eds). *Principles of Cosmetics for the Dermatologist* St. Louis, Mosby, 1982, pp 265-273.
24. Phillips L. A comparison of rabbit and human skin response to certain irritants. *Toxicol Appl Pharmacol* 1972;21:369-382.
25. Lasagna L. Regulatory agencies, drugs, and the pregnant patient, in Stern L (ed). *Drug Use in Pregnancy*. ADES Health, Science Press, 1984.
26. Lewis PJ. Animal tests for teratogenicity, their relevance to clinical practice, in Hawkins DF (ed). *Drugs and Pregnancy: Human Teratogenesis and Related Problems*. Edinburgh, Churchill Livingston, 1983, pp 17-21.
27. Smithells RW. Drug teratogenesis, in Inman WH (ed). *Monitoring for Drug Safety*. Philadelphia, JB Lippincott, 1980.
28. Salsburg D. The lifetime feeding study in mice and rats--an examination of its validity as a bioassay for human carcinogens. *Fundament Appl Toxicol* 1983;3:63-67.
29. Freedman DA, Zeisel H. From mouse to man: The quantitative assessment of cancer risks. Stat Sci 1988;3:3-28.
30. Heywood R. Clinical toxicity--could it have been predicted? Post-market experience, in Lumley CE, Walker SR (eds). *Animal Toxicity Studies: Their Relevance for Man*. Lancaster, Quay Pub, 1989.
31. Hansen RW. The pharmaceutical development process: Estimates of development costs and times and the effects of proposed regulatory changes, in Chien R (ed). *Issues in Pharmaceutical Economics*. DC Health, 1979:151-181.
32. Irwin S. Drug screening and evaluative procedures. *Science* 1962;136:123-128.
33. Hempel CG. *Philosophy of Natural Science*. Englewood Cliffs, NJ, Prentice-Hall, 1966.
34. Popper KR. *The Logic of Scientific Discovery*. New York, Harper, 1968.
35. Root-Bernstein RS. *Discovering*. Cambridge, Harvard Univ Pr, 1989.
36. Reines BP. On the locus of medical discovery. *J Medicine Philosophy* 1991;16:183-209.
37. Reines BP. Psychopharmacologic discovery: The relative contributions of clinical and laboratory studies. *Perspec Med Res* 1990;2:13-26.
38. Beeson PB. The growth of knowledge about a disease: Hepatitis. Am J Med 1979;67: 366-370.
39. Reines BP. On the role of anomaly in Harvey's discovery of the mechanism of the pulse. Perspec Biol Med 1990;34:128-133.
40. Beeson PB. Animals in research: Context of a quote [Letter]. *Science* 1989;245:1437.
41. Good RA. Runestones in immunology. *J Immunol* 1976;117:1413-1428.

42. Good RA. Keystones. *J Clin Invest* 1968;47:1466-1471.
43. Good RA. The value of animal research [letter]. *Science* 1991;
44. Sitaram N, Gershon S. Animal models to clinical testing--promises and pitfalls. *Prog Neuro-psychopharmacol Biol Psychiat* 1983;7:227-228.
45. Sitaram N, Gershon S. Gershon ES. Use of animals in research [letter]. *Am J Psychiat* 1988;145:653.
46. Committee on the Use of Laboratory Animals in Biomedical and Behavioral Research. *Use of Laboratory Animals in Biomedical and Behavioral Research*. Washington, DC, National Academy Press, 1988.
47. Paul JR. *History of Poliomyelitis*. New Haven, Yale University Press, 1971.
48. Wickman I. *Studien über Poliomyelitis acuta; zugleich ein Beitrag zur Kenntnis der Myelitis acuta*. Berlin, Karger, 1905.
49. Wickman I. *Beiträge zur Kenntnis der Heine-Medinschen Krankheit*. Berlin, Karger, 1907.
50. Sabin AB. Statement of Albert B. Sabin, M.D. [before the Subcommittee on Hospitals and Health Care of the Committee on Veterans' Affairs, House of Representatives]. Serial no. 98-48, April 26, 1984.
51. Von Magnus H. Studies on mouse encephalitis virus (TO strain). *Acta Pathologica* 1950;27:605-624, 1951;28:234-257.

The Process of Medical Discovery

Brandon P. Reines

Recently, certain philosophers of science have challenged the ways historians have traditionally described the process of medical discovery. Many historians have tended to provide *descriptive* accounts of medical discovery by focusing on particular successful experiments. Their focus, in general, has been priority disputes or biographical information about principal investigators. Consequently, most medical historians have failed to critically examine the underlying conceptual evolution of medical discoveries.[1] Philosopher Thomas Nickles' *normative* account of discovery in the physical sciences offers a framework for understanding discovery in the life sciences.[2,3] Nickles, seeking to describe the *logic* and *origin* of discovery, traces the evolution of physical discoveries from the initial anomalous observations to later confirmatory laboratory experiments. Nickles argues that the results of experimental manipulations (which can only approximate natural phenomena) can never be directly extrapolated from the lab to the real world. He concludes that discoveries arise from knowledge of existing theory and an ability to interpret, and perceive anomalies in, a broad range of data; significant discoveries rarely derive from an individual experimental effort.

Laboratory testing of theories in the life sciences tends to be even more problematic than in the physical sciences, because it is difficult to reproduce natural phenomena of complex, living organisms in the laboratory. Animal experiments, which involve relatively simple manipulations designed to produce a particular result, provide contrived evidence in support of a particular theory. Researchers have at their disposal a nearly infinite range of experimental manipulations that can be performed on animals of different species, and they can fashion the experimental protocol so that they obtain data that "confirm" a theory actually derived from prior clinical observation and investigation. In reality, laboratory data on other species can neither disprove a hypothesis about humans nor necessitate the formulation of a new hypothesis. Yet, historians of science routinely credit such experimentation, rather than the preceding clinical investigation and hypothesis, as the source of discovery. Consequently, medical historians generally present the animal experimenter as the discoverer and relegate the actual discoverer--the clinician--to anonymity or lesser importance.

Endocrinology

The Adrenal Glands

During the mid-19th century, most physiologists contended that nervous reflexes mediate organic functions--a doctrine known as nervism. The anomalies that eventually discredited this doctrine were clinically observed.

In 1855, physician Thomas Addison described five human cases of tuberculous invasion of the adrenal glands and nearby nervous structures, noting symptoms of anemia, general debilitation, cardiac "feebleness," stomach "irritability," and skin discoloration. Addison hypothesized that the adrenal glands must secrete a substance vital to health.[4]

In an effort to test Addison's hypothesis, experimenters then removed animals' adrenal glands. No experiment reproduced the symptoms of Addison's disease,[5] but researchers were able to induce skin discoloration by experimental bilateral adrenalectomy did induce skin discoloration.[6] Experimental adrenalectomy often caused rapid death of the animals used.[7] Although the researchers attributed the deaths of many of their rat and mice subjects to surgical trauma, many physiologists interpreted the deaths as evidence that the adrenal glands filter harmful toxins from the blood.[8]

In 1882, physician James F. Goodhart first firmly refuted nervism by reporting cases of Addison's disease caused by simple atrophy of the adrenal glands.[9] Addison's hypothesis then received wider acceptance.

In 1893, physician-physiologist George W. Oliver tested the hypothesis that adrenal secretions affect blood pressure, by feeding an adrenal extract to his son (who became somewhat ill).[10] Using a device of his own design, Oliver measured the diameter of the radial artery (in the forearm) and found it to be dramatically decreased. Oliver concluded that the adrenal glands must contain a substance that raises blood pressure by constricting blood vessels. Oliver never stated exactly how he derived the hypothesis, but he must have had a working hypothesis before he gave adrenal extract to his son and measured blood vessel diameter. Otherwise, his experiment on his son seems illogical. Most likely, he was inspired by the low blood pressure seen in Addison's disease.

According to the standard historical account, when Oliver arrived at experimental physiologist Edward A. Shafer's laboratory to test the adrenal extract on animals, a dog was fortuitously hooked to a mercury manometer at the time. The effects of the adrenal extract on blood pressure were noted immediately. The history of medicine literature commonly relates such dramatic, "happy accident" stories, which suggest that discoveries occur in the laboratory. Like many such stories, this one is questionable. Henry H. Dale, who related this account, heard it third-hand, and even he later wrote, "I can find no contemporary record even to suggest what the experiment might have been."[10] Oliver's writings also contradict this account.[11,12] Oliver and Shafer's experiments on animals were not lucky accidents, but well-planned manipulations that must have required forethought. For example, their experiments on dogs involved cutting the dogs' spinal cords and injecting very low doses of adrenal extract into their veins.[13]

Through this highly invasive and contrived procedure, Oliver and Schafer raised the dogs' blood pressure. (Most likely, Oliver and Schafer cut the dogs' spinal cords in order to remove any inhibitory influence of the central nervous system that might have lessened the extract's effect on blood pressure.)

Although Oliver's hypothesis--derived from human investigations--provided the rationale for the experiments on dogs, medical historians have generally credited Schafer with the role of pioneer endocrinologist, highlighting the animal experiments and minimizing the contribution of the observations of humans that preceded them.

The Ovaries

In many ways, discovery of the ovaries' endocrine function paralleled discovery of the adrenal glands' function.

In the 19th century, the influential physiologist Eduard Pfluger asserted that menstruation results from the growing ovum impinging on the ovarian nerves and, by reflex, causing uterine changes.[14] However, in 1895, surgeon Robert T. Morris observed that some women menstruate and become pregnant *after* their ovaries have been surgically removed.[15] (Subsequent post-mortem studies of such women revealed that a small fragment of ovarian tissue had inadvertently been left behind.) In such cases the ovum cannot impinge on the ovarian nerves; therefore, Morris hypothesized that ovarian secretion, not reflex action, must be crucial in inducing menstruation. With this theory in mind, he transplanted ovarian tissue into the uteruses of women unable to menstruate or become pregnant due to prior ovariectomy or reproductive-tract pathology.[16]

According to Morris, researcher Emil Knauer quickly learned of Morris' findings by way of Morris' assistant, Morris Schlapp. Using animal experimentation, Knauer then attempted to mirror Morris' findings. In 1896, Knauer reported that rabbits whose ovaries had been excised and implanted elsewhere in their body did not experience uterine atrophy.[17] He, not Morris, became known as the discoverer of the ovaries' endocrine function.

Angiology and Reconstructive Vascular Surgery

Angiology (the science of blood vessels), which made modern reconstructive vascular surgery possible, also evolved from clinical observation.

The Vascular Endothelium

The healing capacity of the vascular endothelium (the cells comprising blood vessels' innermost layer) underlies surgical repair of blood vessels. In the process of healing, the vascular endothelium forms connective scar tissue.

In the 1880s, pathologist Ernst Ziegler observed that the endothelium of ligated arteries usually forms scar tissue and likened this capacity for repair to that of abdominal lining.[18] Surgeons began to translate their experience with abdominal surgery to vascular surgery.

In aneurysm surgery, Robert Abbe and others tested whether arteries have an inner lining capable of forming scar tissue.[19] These surgeons irritated arteries' inner lining (for example, with a surgical needle) in the hope of stimulating reparative processes, and this appeared to improve surgical results.[20]

Vascular Anastomosis

In the 1890s, as surgeons were discovering that arteries are lined by cells with a capacity for active repair, they hypothesized the possibility of performing vascular anastomosis (reuniting the two severed ends of a blood vessel).[21] Morris then attempted the procedure in rabbits. The effort failed, apparently because of resulting infections.[21] Nevertheless, Morris suggested the procedure to surgeon James B. Murphy.

In 1897, Murphy published the first report on vascular anastomosis in human patients.[22] The procedure was not entirely successful--partly because of post-surgical infection, partly because Murphy inserted one severed end of the blood vessel into the other rather than aligning them so that the two ends' inner linings could adhere to each other.[23] Nevertheless, Murphy's partially successful clinical cases influenced both clinical and laboratory investigators of vascular anastomosis, including Alexis Carrel.[24]

In 1912, Carrel won the Nobel Prize for his method of vascular anastomosis; the method, he stated, "came into existence nine years ago from the study of the technique of [physician] Payr and of Murphy."[25] Carral claimed to develop the principle using human cadavers and two living dogs.

Although Carrel and his animal research colleague Stephen Watts first demonstrated the advisability of suturing blood vessels inner lining to inner lining in nonhuman animals, their work's guiding hypothesis derived from the clinical research of surgeons, such as Abbe, who were repairing arteries with aneurysms.

Veins' Tolerance of Arterial Blood Pressure

In 1728, William Hunter first reported an arteriovenous aneurysm, an abnormal connection between an artery and a vein that introduces blood into venous circulation under unnaturally high pressure.[26]

Nearly two centuries later, surgeon Alejandro San Martin y Satrustigui analyzed cases of arteriovenous aneurysm and concluded that, because the vein abnormally connected to an artery pulsates throughout the patient's life, veins must be able to withstand the high blood pressure characteristic of arteries. San Martin hypothesized the possibility of using grafted veins as substitutes for portions of damaged arteries.[27,28]

San Martin suggested to his student José Goyanes that he attempt to connect two cut ends of an artery by means of a venous graft. In 1906, following San Martin's advice, Goyanes excised an aneurysm and replaced it with a segment of nearby vein.[27] The patient fared well. Goyanes' success encouraged other surgeons to use vein grafts to repair arterial segments.

The Bypass Principle

In 1948, French surgeon Jean Kunlin performed the first bypass operation.[29] Confronted with arterial blockage in a patient's leg, Kunlin reasoned that the chance of saving the leg might be improved if the section of blocked artery were left intact rather than excised, since excision would destroy smaller blood vessels that formed collaterals around the damaged section of artery and the collateral circulation such vessels provide. And so, Kunlin grafted one of the patient's own saphenous veins around the blockage. American surgeons quickly appreciated the principle of preserving collateral circulation.

However, the principle of grafting a patient's own vein remained largely ignored well into the 1960s. Although surgeons at Walter Reed Army Hospital successfully used autovein grafting in the early 1950s,[30] most surgeons opted instead for arterial grafts. According to vascular surgeons Rodolfo Domingo, Charles C. Fries, Philip N. Sawyer, and Sigmund A. Wesolowski, the general bias against using a patient's own vein for bypass surgery resulted from experimental findings in animals that veins engrafted in the arterial system often underwent aneurysmal dilatation (ballooning of a blood vessel due to increased pressure).[31] Nevertheless, by repeatedly performing clinical bypass surgery of leg arteries, W. Andrew Dale, Robert Linton, Gregory Mavor, and others demonstrated the success of bypass surgery using a patient's saphenous vein.[32,33]

Hematology

Red-Blood-Cell Groups

In 1900, hematologist Karl Landsteiner proposed the existence of A, B, and O human red-blood-cell groups as the explanation for transfusion reactions between human beings.[34] The validity of grouping blood types into A, B, and O was supported by *in vitro* assays of human sera and red blood cells and confirmed by the effectiveness of using blood typing to prevent transfusion reactions.

Rh Factor

In 1939, hematologist Philip Levine first hypothesized the existence of a third antigen (a substance that induces antibody production), in addition to A and B antigens, on the surface of human red blood cells.[35] Levine's hypothesis was prompted by the case of a woman who gave birth to a severely decomposed fetus that had been dead for several months: when the woman was subsequently transfused with her husband's ABO-matched blood, she suffered a severe reaction. Levine reasoned that the mother, due to prolonged exposure to the fetus, must have already produced antibodies to some antigen present in both the fetus's and the father's blood. That is, some previously unknown red-blood-cell antigen must have been responsible for the mother's immune response. Levine did not, however, name this newly hypothesized antigen.[36]

Landsteiner and hematologist Alexander Wiener soon dubbed the antigen "Rh (rhesus) factor."[37] When, in *in vitro* tests, the blood serum of humans who had shown an adverse reaction to ABO-matched blood was mixed with human red blood cells of compatible type, about 80% of samples showed clumping of red blood cells due to antibody attachment in response to an antigen. In similar tests the blood serum of rabbits who had been injected (in Landsteiner and Wiener's laboratory) with red blood cells from rhesus monkeys and had produced antibodies in reaction to rhesus red-blood-cell antigens *also* showed about 80% clumping when mixed with human red blood cells.[38] The misnomer "Rh factor" was based on this finding that rabbits produce an antibody to some rhesus red-blood-cell antigen that also reacts to a human red-blood-cell antigen.

Levine then attempted to confirm his own theory by replicating Landsteiner and Wiener's experimental results; having failed to do so, in 1961, Levine asserted that the rhesus-monkey antigen identified by Landsteiner and Wiener must differ from the human one.[39]

Levine's theory explained the pathogenesis of erythroblastosis fetalis ("rhesus disease of the newborn"), in which an Rh-negative mother produces antibodies against the Rh factor in the blood of an Rh-positive fetus, thereby destroying the fetus' red blood cells.[40] Nevertheless, Wiener is generally given more credit for the discovery of Rh factor and its relationship to disease than Levine, even though Landsteiner and Wiener's Rh experiments never elucidated any human disease.

White-Blood-Cell Groups

Initially white-blood-cell groups were investigated with the hope of improving the success of tissue and organ transplants. In the 1950s clinical investigators such as Jean Dausett, Jan J. van Rood, and Rose Payne began exploring human white-cell groups.[41-43] Because transfusion reactions occurred despite careful typing by all known human red-cell antigens, these investigators hypothesized the existence of previously unidentified white-cell antigens. They then used *in vitro* immunological tests to further characterize those antigens.

By 1948, animal experimenters such as Peter Gorer and George Snell had concluded that a specific group of genes determines which antigens are present on a mouse's cells and, therefore, which cells transplanted from another mouse will provoke an immune response to foreign antigens. They called the group of genes the "major histocompatibility complex" (MHC).[44,45] In the mouse, the MHC became known as the histocompatibility-2 (H-2) system.

While determining the human white-cell groups through studies of human patients, clinical investigators attempted to relate their findings to MHC theory--even contending, as of 1965, that they were uncovering the "human MHC"--thereby obscuring their discoveries' clinical origins.[46]

By the late 1960s, however, H-2 researchers had developed so elaborate an explanation of their laboratory findings that one of these researchers, Jan Klein, recalls: "The H-2 system was often considered an exotic curiosity completely detached from reality."[47] In contrast, clinical investigators developed a simple two-locus framework by which to interpret the white-cell data.

In 1966, Walter Bodmer, Payne, and colleagues argued that the HL-A histocompatibility complex of humans is composed of two distinct series, which they labeled A and B.[48] Snell and Erik Thorsby then maintained that the mouse H-2 framework should be simplified to reflect two main loci (K and D) analogous to the human A and B loci.[49] Thorsby wrote, "Based on serological and genetic evidence from the HL-A system, a tentative new H-2 model of two segregant series is suggested."[49] Yet, knowledge of human histocompatibility is generally attributed to the mouse research of Snell, Gorer, and their co-workers.

Conclusion

Historians have generally failed to recognize the clinical origins of medical discovery. Routinely, medical discoveries derived from observation of clinicopathologic anomalies are attributed to laboratory experimentation. Because of species differences in anatomy and physiology, extrapolation (by analogy) from laboratory to clinical phenomena is, at best, unreliable.

References

1. Reines BP. On the locus of medical discovery. *The Journal of Medicine and Philosophy* 1991;16:183-209.
2. Nickles T. Justification and experiment, in Gooding D, Pinch T (eds). *The Uses of Experiment*. Cambridge, University Press, 1989, pp 299-333.
3. Nickles T. Beyond divorce: Current status of the discovery debate. *Philosophy of Science*

1985;552:177-206.

4. Addison T. *On the Constitutional and Local Effects of Disease of the Suprarenal Capsules*. London, Samuel Highley, 1855.
5. Brown-Sequard CE. Recherches experimentales sur la physiologie et al pathologie des capsules surrenales. *Arch Gen Med* 1856;8:385-401, 572-598.
6. Tizzoni G. Sur la physio-pathologie des capsules surrenales. *Arch Ital Biol* 1884;5:333-340.
7. Harley G. An experimental inquiry into the function of the supra-renal capsules and their supposed connection with bronzed skin. *British and Foreign Medical-Chirurgical Review* 1858;21:204-221, 498-510.
8. de Domenicis N. Pourquoi l'extirpation des capsules surrenales amene la mort chez les animaux. *Arch Physiol* 1894;6:810-815.
9. Goodhart J. Simple atrophy of the supra-renal capsules, accompanied by melasmasupra-renale and other symptoms of Addison's disease. *Trans Path Soc London* 1882;33:340-345.
10. Dale HH. Accident and opportunism in medical research. *Br Med J* 1948;2:451-455.
11. Oliver G. *Pulse Gauging: A Clinical Study of Radial Measurement and Pulse-Pressure*. London, HK Lewis, 1895.
12. Oliver G. A contribution to the study of the blood and circulation. *Br Med J* 1896;1:1374-1377.
13. Oliver G, Shafer E. On the physiological action of extract of the suprarenal capsules. *J Physiol* 1894;17:i-v.
14. Simmer H. Pfluger's nerve reflex theory of menstruation: The product of analogy, teleology and neurophysiology. *Clio Medica* 1977;12:57-90.
15. Morris RT. The ovarian graft. *New York Med J* 1895;62:436-437.
16. Morris RT. Notes on ovarian grafting. *Medical Record* 1901;59:83-87.
17. Knauer E. Einige versuche uber ovarientransplantation bei kaninchen. *Centrablatt fur Gynakologie* 1896;20:524-528.
18. Ziegler E. *A Textbook of General Pathological Anatomy and Pathogenesis*. New York, Wood Pub, 1883-1887.
19. Abbe R. Aneurysmorrhaphy: Personal experience with the modern method of treating aneurysm. *Ann Surg* 1908;48:10-15.
20. Morris RT. The serous coat of blood vessels compared with the peritoneum. *Ann Surg* 1908;48:18-21.
21. Morris RT. *Fifty Years A Surgeon*. New York, EP Dutton, 1935.
22. Murphy JB. Resection of arteries and veins injured in continuity. *Med Record* 1897:51:73-88.
23. Stewart FT. End-to-end anastomosis of the brachial artery [discussion]. *Ann Surg* 1908;48:152-155.
24. Carrel A. Technique and remote results of vascular anastomoses. *Surg Gynecol Obstet* 1912;14:246-250.
25. Watts S. The suture of blood vessels. Implantation and transplantation of vessels and organs. An historical and experimental study. *Bull Johns Hopkins Hospital* 1907;18:154-192.
26. Hunter W. XXXVI Further observations on a particular species of aneurysm. *Medical Observation Society of the Physicians of London* 1761;2:390-414.
27. Goyanes J. Substitution plastica de las arterias por las venas, o arterioplastica venosa, aplicada, como nuevo metodo, al tratamiento de los aneurismas. *El Siglio Medico*

1906;346.

28. Goyanes J. San Martin and his work [lecture at Athenaem of Madrid, December 1920]. Academy of the R.A.N. of Medicine, 1920.
29. Kunlin J. The treatment of arterial obstruction by vein grafting. *Arch Mal Coeur* 1949;42:371-375.
30. Cooke FN, Hughes CW, Jahnke EJ, Seeley SF. Homologous arterial grafts and autogenous vein grafts used to bridge large arterial defects in man: A report on fourteen cases. *Surgery* 1953;33:183-189.
31. Domingo RT, Fries CC, Sawyer PN, Wesolowski SA. Peripheral arterial reconstruction: Transplantation of autologous veins. *Trans Am Soc Artificial Internal Organs* 1963;IX: 305-308.
32. Mavor G. Autogenous vein grafts, in Mackey WA (ed). *Arterial Surgery*. New York, MacMillan, 1964.
33. Dale WA, DeWeese JA, Merle Scott WJ. Autogenous venous shunt grafts: Rational and report of 31 for atherosclerosis. *Surgery* 1959;46:145-161.
34. Landsteiner K. Uber agglutinationserscheinungen normalen menschlichen blutes. *Wien Klin Wschr* 1901;14:1132-1135.
35. Levine P, Stetson RE. An unusual case of intra-group agglutination. *JAMA* 1939;113: 126-127.
36. Zimmerman D. *Rh: The Intimate History of a Disease and its Conquest*. New York, MacMillan, 1973.
37. Landsteiner K, Wiener AS. An agglutinable factor in human blood recognized by immune sera for rhesus blood. *Proc Soc Exp Biol Med* 1940;43:223-224.
38. Wiener AS. Karl Landsteiner, MD: History of the Rh-Hr blood group system. *NY State J Med* 1969;69:2915-2935.
39. Levine P. The discovery of Rh hemolytic disease. *Vox Sanguis* 1984;47:187-190.
40. Levine P. The influence of the ABO system on Rh hemolytic disease. *Human Biology* 1958;30:14-20.
41. Dausset J, Nenna A. Presence d'une leuco-agglutinine dans le serum d'un cas d'agranulocytose chronique. *CR Society for Biology* 1952:140:1534-1536.
42. Payne R. Leukocyte agglutinins in human sera. *Arch Int Med* 1957;99:587-591.
43. van Rood JJ, Eernisse JG, van Leeuwen A. Leucocyte antibodies in sera from pregnant women. *Nature* 1958;181:1735-1736.
44. Snell GD. Histocompatibility genes of the mouse II. Production and analysis of isogenic resistant lines. *J Nat Canc Inst* 1958;21:843-848.
45. Gorer P. The detection of antigenic differences in mouse erythocytes by the employment of immune sera. *Br J Exp Biol* 1936;17:42-46.
46. Dausett J, Ivanyi P, Ivanyi D. Tissue antigens in humans. Identification of a complex system (Hu-1), in Dausett J (ed). *Histocompatability testing 1965*. Copenhagen, Munksgaard, 1965.
47. Klein J. *Biology of the Mouse Histocompatability-2 Complex* [Chapter 1, History]. New York, Springer-Verlag, 1975.
48. Bodmer W, Bodmer J, Adler S, Payne S, Bialek J. Genetics of 4 and LA human leukocyte groups. *Ann NY Acad Sci* 1966;129:473-489.
49. Thorsby E. A tentative new model for the organization of the mouse H-2 histocompatability system: Two segregant series of antigens. *Eur J Immunol* 1971;1:57-59.

Edward H. Ahrens, Jr. *The Crisis in Clinical Research: Overcoming Institutional Obstacles*.

Oxford University Press, New York, 1992.

This provocative analysis of U.S. research funding documents a dramatic decline in patient-centered basic research on human physiology and pathology. Physician and clinical researcher Edward H. Ahrens, Jr. argues that "basic research" (the study of disease mechanisms) has shifted from the clinic to the laboratory, and this shift threatens to undermine research productivity. Ahrens provides thorough statistical evidence and political analyses of the factors that have contributed to this trend.

Ahrens reviews trends in the U.S. While the National Institutes of Health (NIH) budget constituted 41% of U.S. health R&D in 1979, the percentage dropped to 34% by 1988. Similarly, support for health R&D from other federal agencies fell from 19% in 1979 to 12% in 1988. However, industry support increased from 29% in 1979 to 41% in 1988. Also, in constant 1979 dollars, total health R&D substantially increased--from $7.133 billion in 1979 to $18.729 billion in 1988. Although the 1991 NIH budget constituted only 3.8% of non-defense discretionary spending, this percentage has been growing annually by 6.7% since 1981.

Despite increased federal dollars for health R&D, the percentage of proposed projects awarded NIH grants has somewhat declined. From 1976 to 1988, 31% of all NIH grant applications resulted in funding; in 1989 the figure was 27.5%. Factors that contributed to slightly heightened competition for grants include increases in the number of investigators and in research costs. Direct costs (the expenses of individual research projects) rose more than sevenfold from 1970 to 1988, while indirect costs (expenses incurred by the principal investigator's institution for such research overhead as building maintenance) rose almost fourfold. Indirect costs averaged 46% of direct costs, ranging from about 8% for training grants to 65% or more for research preformed at major medical centers.

From 1976 to 1988, MDs acting as principal investigators had a success rate of 31% for initial grant application. Seven percent were successful upon second submission (most unsuccessful grant applications are resubmitted), and 8% of grants succeeded on the third to fifth submission. PhDs had virtually the same success rates: 31%, 8%, and 8%, respectively. Medical schools, however, significantly varied in their success rates. The top 40 medical schools had approximately 40% grant-application success, while the bottom 40 had only about 20% success.

Of extramural NIH awards, 52% went to U.S. medical schools and their affiliated hosptials. Non-federal research institutes (both non-profit and for-profit) and hospitals not affiliated with medical schools received 25% of the grant money, while schools of arts and sciences received 12%, public health and dental schools received 7%, and other institutions of higher education received 4%.

Ahrens examines the funding disparities between different types of research, particularly between "basic patient-oriented research" (basic POR) and other types of research that Ahrens also designates as "clinical." In Ahrens' terminology, basic POR studies the *mechanisms* of human disease in human patients; other "clinical" research includes applied POR--which studies the *management* of human disease (e.g., clinical drug trials, studies of preventive strategies)--*in vitro* research on materials of human origin, and "animal models" of human health and disease. Ahrens acknowledges, however, that the clinical relevance of animal models is controversial: "There is not now, nor theoretically will there ever be, a perfect animal model for any of the major human diseases." (p. 177) Despite their dubious utility, animal models of human diseases received, during the decade 1977-1987, more NIH grant money than any other research method--27.2% of all NIH extramural funding.

Ahrens' principal concern is the rapid decline in financial support for basic POR. Whereas this research "dominated the pages of clinical research publications and the annual meetings of clinical investigators" in the 1950s and 60s, "the pendulum has swung decidedly toward bench research [reductionist, "controlled" laboratory research that focuses on narrowly focussed aspects of a problem]. . . and away from Basic to Applied POR" (pp. 111-112). In a random review of recently funded grant proposals, Ahrens found that fewer than 8% of the projects were in the area of basic POR.

Why does basic POR have difficulty competing with other types of research for NIH funds? According to Ahrens, for one thing, basic POR researchers often have difficulty recruiting patients who faithfully adhere to the research protocol. Also, unlike those who experiment on animals, POR investigators are constrained by the requirement that protocols be acceptable to human-subject review boards. In general, too, basic POR is more costly than other types of health research. Reasons for this include costs of patient recruitment, hospitalization expenses, and the lenghty duration of many clinical research projects due to the long natural histories of many human diseases.

In addition to these factors, the composition of NIH grant review committees often has the effect of discouraging basic POR, since these committees are generally comprised of scientists and physicians who favor laboratory research. Increasingly, Ahrens says, funding decisions are based on a project's likelihood of producing publishable results, rather than its actual scientific merit. He notes that many laboratory researchers, "lacking familiarity with POR, believe that POR facilities exist simply to act as the final step in translating flashes of genius of laboratory scientists into clinical reality. . . . In fact, this has happened only rarely. During my 40 years at the Rockefeller Hospital, I recall only one instance in which a laboratory investigation by biochemists was turned into a testable hypothesis in patients--namely, the treatment of sickle-cell crisis with cyanate." (p. 146)

Basic POR investigators also face deterrents within their own academic institutions. Under increasing financial pressure, many medical centers have made income generation the priority. Since services to patients readily generate income, physicians who would otherwise conduct POR research are often required to spend most of their time providing these services.

Advocating the restoration of balance to U.S. health research, Ahrens recommends more unrestricted training grants to encourage young POR scientists, even if this means less funds available for specific research projects. Also, he proposes designating special grant-review committees to consider basic POR projects only, so that these projects will not compete directly with those representing other research approaches.

Ahrens argues forcefully that basic patient-centered research is vital and that the declining support for this research could seriously undermine medical progress.

Stephen R. Kaufman, M.D.

Michael Balls, James Bridges, Jacqueline Southee (eds.) *Animals and Alternatives in Toxicology: Present Status and Future Prospects.*

VCH Publishers, New York, 1991.

This book presents the proceedings of a conference held in November of 1990 at the Royal College of Physicians in London. Conferees discussed the Second Report of the Fund for Replacement of Animals in Medical Experiments (FRAME) Toxicity Committee. The nineteen prominent toxicologists who comprise the Committee had formed twelve working parties to investigate specific topics. Thirty additional leaders of the toxicology community had input to the working parties, helping them to assess the prospects for decreasing or eliminating animal testing and develop recommendations for minimizing animal use and suffering.

Most working parties of toxicologists acknowledged that current animal tests are inadequate. However, most were not optimistic that non-animal methods would completely replace animal tests in the near future. Most working parties concluded, on scientific as well as animal welfare grounds, that toxicity tests need improvement. According to Andre McLean, considerable progress has been made, but there is work to be done:

> Great advances in various databases mean that computer searches are accessible to everyone. . . . unquestionably, our power of intellectual analysis has improved enormously. Against that, our use of animals in toxicology appears very crude and old-fashioned -- sometimes because we haven't yet got an alternative, but sometimes because we have not thought of how to do things a different way. . . . The idea that the regulators should still demand out-of-date, useless, scientifically-invalid, hopeless studies, which involve animals, is a scandal at the political level, which to a considerable extent is out of our [toxicologists'] direct control. (p. 342)

Although some conference participants seemed unduly reluctant to recommend significant change, the proceedings do provide a thorough analysis of the scientific strengths and weaknesses of animal and non-animal tests.

Kathryn Hahner, Ph.D.

Irwin D. Bross. *Scientific Fraud vs. Scientific Truth.*

Biomedical Metatechnology Press, Eggertsville, New York, 1991.

In this collection of case studies, Irwin Bross details how "Official Science" bureaucrats use fraudulent "scientific" data to defend political policy. Bross--who has co-authored over 350 scientific papers, has been involved in the major clinical trials of many cancer treatments, and has worked within the scientific establishment for years--develops the thesis, "The establishment is the enemy of the enterprise."

Most research scientists, Bross argues, genuinely pursue truth, but science administrators reach positions of prominence because of their political loyalties. The politicians who appoint these administrators are beholden to the wealthy industry concerns that underwrite their campaigns. Science administrators are puppets of big business, and "science" itself is a public relations tool that provides "evidence" (often fraudulent) to support industry's positions.

For example, science administrators continue to advocate high-dose radiation tests on animals as a (supposed) means of establishing limits of "safe" low-dose radiation exposure (such as that occurring during X-ray tests) even though the high-dose animal data cannot be extrapolated to low-dose human exposure. The nuclear industry uses the inaccurate and invalid animal data to defend itself against evidence of increased cancer incidence near nuclear power plants; the Department of Defense uses the data to defend itself against disability claims by cancer-stricken veterans exposed to nuclear bomb tests during the 1950s.

In *Scientific Fraud vs. Scientific Truth* Bross expands on themes he has discussed in such earlier works as *Crimes of Official Science; A Casebook* (1987) and *Scientific Strategies to Save Your Life* (1981). He updates readers on the Love Canal controversy, involving a continuing misinformation campaign by Official Science. He also argues, as he has for years, that routine mammography *increases* a woman's risk of breast cancer. Bross' claim has been strengthened by a recent Canadian study in which women who received routine mammographies had a 52% greater rate of death from breast cancer than women who did not.

Bross' evidence that top science administrators have, for decades, intentionally deceived the public is compelling. He encourages grass-roots campaigns aimed at increasing the public's scientific literacy; public ignorance, he maintains, allows "scientific" misinformation to flourish. Bross suggests zero-budgeting the NIH, which he considers thoroughly corrupt, and instituting a decentralized scientific enterprise comprised of independent clinical researchers dedicated to truth and public health.

Stephen R. Kaufman, M.D.

Reitman, Judith. *Stolen for Profit: How the Medical Establishment is Funding a National Pet-Theft Conspiracy.*

New York, Pharos Books, 1992.

A dog or cat owner's worst nightmare is that their beloved companion might end up a research subject. Investigative reporter Judith Reitman thoroughly documents that this has been the fate of millions of "lost" and stolen pets. The animal-research industry has created a lucrative market for "random-source" dogs, paying up to $300-550 for large dogs. Unlike purpose-bred dogs, former pets are "ideal" research subjects because they are accustomed to human interaction and unlikely to resist or bite during frightening or painful procedures.

Reitman focuses on a recent Los Angeles criminal case in which a ring of dealers was found guilty of pet theft. Responding to "Free To A Good Home" ads in local papers, the dealers claimed to be interested in adopting pets but actually sold them to labs, including Cedars Sinai, Loma Linda, and the Veteran's Hospital in Sepulveda.

The problem of pet theft extends well beyond one local network, however. Reitman details numerous episodes nationwide in which entire neighborhoods have had dogs disappear over a short period. One lab sought to obtain 126 German Shorthaired Pointers within six weeks. Mary Warner of Action 81, a grassroots organization that monitors and documents pet theft, has commented, "Where did the researchers from the lab expect to get [them]? Well, residents near the lab soon found out."

Large-scale, organized pet theft would be impossible if the U.S. Department of Agriculture enforced existing legislation. Reitman documents how key USDA administrators have impeded efforts to regulate lab animal acquisition. A network of "bunchers" (those who collect animals, often through theft or false representation, for sale to licensed dealers), dealers, and local law-enforcement officials prevents pet owners from locating their lost animals, while USDA officials look the other way. Research institutions claim that, to the best of their knowledge, they do not purchase stolen animals. However, they generally bar pet owners from entering lab-animal facilities to search for lost companions, and many purchase from dealers who routinely falsify records, listing non-existent or long deceased persons as those who supply them with dogs and cats.

Not surprisingly, the pet-theft network treats the animals abusively. Bunchers and dealers, for example, regularly handle animals in the most brutal manner, as well as transport and hold them under grossly inhumane conditions. Still research institutions continue to do business with the pet-theft network and are unlikely to be swayed by animal welfare concerns. (The animal research industry has affiliated with organizations such as Putting People First, that openly derides concern for animals.)

Reitman documents her arguments conclusively. However, not totally convincing is her evidence regarding a 1992 report that concluded that the animal-research industry is not primarily responsible for the stolen pet problem, although it does contribute heavily. Reitman suggests that a foundation with weak ties to the animal-research industry influenced the contents of a report prepared by the *Animals' Agenda*, prompting the animal rights magazine to minimize the animal research industry's complicity in the stolen pet trade. In general, Reitman's book does offer abundant evidence that the animal-research industry and the medical establishment are integrally involved with the stolen pet trade.

Stephen R. Kaufman, M.D.

Committee on the Use of Animals in Research. *Science, Medicine, and Animals.*

National Academy Press, Washington, D.C., 1991.

With the professed purpose of informing the debate on animal research, the Committee on the Use of Animals at the National Academy of Sciences (NAS) has produced the booklet *Science, Medicine, and Animals*, aimed at the general public. In reality, the Committee has produced a one-sided document that uncritically endorses animal experimentation. By dismissing animal rights as a dangerous minority viewpoint and failing to provide a fair, accurate explanation of the concept, the booklet avoids addressing legitimate moral concerns about animal research. Similarly, this document avoids addressing valid scientific objections to animal experimentation by never so much as acknowledging the growing criticism from within scientific circles.

In a manner of presentation that favors vague generalization over specific evidence, the booklet ranges from cancer and heart disease to psychology research and control of infectious diseases to pound seizure and animal rights. Even those sections that include detailed discussions omit crucial facts. For example, one section mentions a lymphoma patient who was cured by chemotherapeutic agents allegedly discovered in mice; while describing the disease and treatment in some detail, the section fails to identify the drugs used. Thus, the claim that these agents were developed through animal studies can be neither verified nor disproved.

Similarly, the booklet claims that "surgical procedures, pain relievers, psychoactive drugs, medications for blood pressure . . . all have been developed and tested in animals." Again, the authors fail to identify the specific measures--thereby preventing focused analysis or dispute of their implication that animal testing contributed to the development of these measures.

Like many other documents that promote animal research, this publication falsely equates *animal testing* with *discovery through animal research*. Though virtually every therapeutic procedure in the last decades has been tested on animals, this is certainly not the same as assuming that these procedures were discovered in animal studies. In fact, careful examination of medical history suggests that medical discovery generally does *not* involve animal experimentation.[1]

Using this false equation of testing with discovery, the NAS report credits animal experimentation with the discovery of chlorpromazine's antipsychotic properties. In truth, chlorpromazine's antipsychotic effect was discovered in human, not animal, studies. A European pharmacology panel has concluded:

> Many valuable drugs (e.g., chlorpromazine as a tranquilizer, imipramine as an antidepressant, beta-adrenoreceptor blocking agents as antihypertensives) have been discovered by observation of their effects in patients suffering from the condition in question. None of these established drugs would have been put forward initially for evaluation for these indications if prediction of therapeutic effect from animals had been mandatory before clinical use. Even with hindsight, some of their valuable effects still have not been shown in animal experiments.[3]

So, while chlorpromazine was indeed *tested* on animals, it was by no means *discovered* in animal studies.

Another case in point is the discovery of AZT's anti-HIV properties, which the booklet attributes to work with primate models of AIDS. In fact, AZT's ability to inhibit HIV replication was first demonstrated in 1985 using a T4-lymphocyte culture infected with the virus.[4] Several weeks later, AZT underwent clinical trials, although no animal tests to show its efficacy had been conducted. The National Cancer Institute researchers who discovered AZT's anti-HIV action have written: "Thus, AZT, a drug chosen on the basis of its selective *in vitro* antiviral effect against HTLV-III [HIV] has been shown to confer a clinical benefit in patients with advanced disease."[5] As mandated by law, AZT was tested on animals; the *discovery* of its anti-HIV properties, however, did not come as a result of animal experimentation.

Even the authors' assertion that animal toxicity testing helps promote safety is disputable.[6-8] Animal toxicity studies commonly yield misleading and contradictory results. In fact, approximately 90% of drugs fail human clinical trials *after* passing animal tests--primarily because they produce adverse reactions in humans.[9] Emerging non-animal methodologies provide a prospect for better, more accurate results. For instance, bone-marrow suppression is a common human adverse reaction to non-steroidal anti-inflammatory agents, but this effect is not predicted by animal studies.[8] In contrast, human granulopoiesis culture can predict this serious adverse drug reaction and even provide a semi-quantitative assessment of the risk.[10]

Since the NAS booklet fails to acknowledge *any* case of animal experimentation's inefficacy, there is good reason to conclude that it was intentionally written as propaganda. The authors' statement, "It makes no sense to sacrifice future human health and well being by not using animals in research today," demonstrates the use of unrestrained hyperbole that pervades the publication. Such emotional hyperbole is particularly unworthy when it emanates from an organization charged with advancing science, which rests on scrupulous avoidance of claims not securely founded on evidence. The public, whose tax dollars help fund the NAS, has much cause to complain.

1. Reines BP. On the locus of medical discovery. *J Med Phil* 1991;16:183-209.

2. Reines BP. Psychopharmacologic discovery: The relative contributions of clinical and laboratory studies. *Perspec Med Res* 1990;2:13-26.

3. Anon. Towards a more rational regulation of the development of new medicines; Report of a European Workshop held in Sestri Levante, Italy, Sep. 28-30, 1976. *Europ J Pharmacol* 1977;11:233-238.

4. Mitsuya H, Weinhold KJ, Furman PA, et al. 3'-Azido-3'-Deoxythymidine (BW A509U): An antiviral agent that inhibits the infectivity and cytopathic effect of human T-lymphotropic virus type III/lymphadenopathy-associated virus *in vitro*. *Proc Natl Acad Sci USA* 1985;82: 7096-7100.

5. Mitsuya H, Broder S. Strategies for antiviral therapy in AIDS. *Nature* 1987;325:773-778.

6. Weatherall M. An end to the search for new drugs? *Nature* 1982;296:387-390.
7. Rang HP, Dale MM. *Pharmacology*. London, Churchill Livingstone, 1987.
8. Heywood R. Clinical toxicity - could it have been predicted? Post-marketing experience, in Lumley CE, Walker SR (eds). *Animal Toxicity Studies: Their Relevance for Man*. Britain, Quay Publishing, 1990, pp 57-67.
9. Levine RR. *Pharmacology: Drug Actions and Reactions*. Boston, Little, Brown & Co, 1978, pp 406-407.
10. Gillian ML, Williams JRB. The effects of some non-steroidal anti-inflammatory drugs on human granulopoiesis *in vitro*. *ATLA* 1985;13:38-47.

Nir Shalev

Medical Research Modernization Committee

The MRMC is comprised of health care professionals who lend their training, experience, and expertise to evaluate the medical and/or scientific merit of research modalities in order to identify archaic methods and to promote sensible, reliable, and efficient methods of research.

MRMC Publications:

* *Perspectives on Animal Research*, volume 1, 1989

The contents include evaluation of learned helplessness research, physiological psychology research, head injury research on cats, amblyopia research on cats, mathematical models, and use of animals in veterinary education. (All volumes are $10; $5 for MRMC members)

* *Perspectives on Animal Research*, volume 1 supplement, 1989.

This special edition features a 134-page review of ten randomly chosen animal models of human diseases.

* *Perspectives on Medical Research*, volume 2, 1990.

The contents include animal models of spinal cord injuries, the process of psychopharmacologic discovery, spheroid cell cultures, the Baby Fae story, and a critique of experiments on the "Silver Spring monkeys."

* *Perspectives on Medical Research*, volume 3, 1991.

The contents include animal models of muscular dystrophy, animal models of degenerative neurological diseases, animal research in psychology, and a critique of the Comroe and Dripps report on the value of basic research.

* *A Critical Look at Animal Experimentation*

This pamphlet summarizes MRMC's concerns about the value of animal models. ($2.40; free for MRMC members)

* *MRMC Report* -- quarterly newsletter (free to MRMC members)

MRMC membership is $25 per year, $10 for students and residents.